DESIGNATED FAT GIRL

DESIGNATED FAT GIRL

A Memoir

Jennifer Joyner

Guilford, Connecticut

To buy books in quantity for corporate use
or incentives, call **(800) 962-0973**
or e-mail **premiums@GlobePequot.com**.

Skirt! is an imprint of Globe Pequot Press.

Skirt! is a registered trademark of Morris Book Publishing, LLC.

Designed by: Sheryl P. Kober
Layout artist: Joanna Beyer
Project manager: Kristen Mellitt

Library of Congress Cataloging-in-Publication Data is available on file.

978-0-7627-5962-0

Printed in the United States of America

10 9 8 7 6 5 4 3 2 1

For Emma & Eli,
Michael & Mom

Contents

Prologue

It is December 2006, and it is actually a pretty good day. For the first time in quite a while, I'm not obsessing every minute of every hour about when and what I will eat next. I have somehow convinced myself to take the day's events as they come—to finally give myself a break—and the freedom in that is exhilarating. I actually notice and enjoy my surroundings. I take an extra moment to play on the floor with my one-year-old son, Eli. He is just starting to walk, and it's fun to watch his face as he attempts steps, his brow furrowed as he tries to figure out his next move. I stop in the middle of getting dressed to read a story to my almost three-year-old daughter, Emma, something I never do because I'm always in such a rush in the morning. I hum a little to myself as I drive the kids to preschool. I stop to appreciate all the Christmas decorations as I travel through the neighborhood. And after school drop-off, I decide to do a little shopping in my favorite children's boutique, something that always makes me smile. *It is a good day.*

As I stand in line to pay for my purchases, I chat with the owner of the store. She is mostly retired, but she hangs out to have something to do, and I've talked with her several times on my near-weekly visits. I ask her if she sells waterproof bed-sheets—I am desperately trying to get Emma potty trained before she turns three, and my mother has suggested I go cold-turkey on the diapers, even at night. The store owner shares with me her theories on potty training, having raised three kids of her own and watched her many grandchildren grow up. She advises me to not force the issue, that Emma will use the potty when she is ready. "Just like you'll lose weight when you're ready," she adds matter-of-factly.

I feel like a sledgehammer has scored a direct hit on my apparently bulging stomach. I open my mouth to speak, but I have to suck in air immediately, my breathlessness saving me from firing back against this poor woman, who is probably only trying to be helpful. She has no idea that for once I'm having a good day—for once I'm not torturing myself about my weight and about food. She doesn't realize she has just brought reality crashing down on me, leaving shards of self-loathing and revulsion slicing me into a million pieces. I don't trust my voice, so I just nod and smile faintly. Mercifully she gives me a knowing smile and pats my arm as she walks away.

I don't remember paying for my stuff—I check out at the register in a daze and then head to my car. At the McDonald's down the street, I attempt to stuff down the incredible pain and sorrow. *This was going to be a good day,* I tell myself. It's hard to cry and eat at the same time, so I choose to eat. Like I always do.

∾

In the grand scheme of things, this wasn't a huge embarrassment. In my many years of battling obesity and morbid obesity, I have suffered much worse in terms of pain and humiliation. But this event sticks out in my mind for two reasons. First, it speaks to how very public a battle with weight is. When you are fat, you can hide from no one, everyone knows you have a problem; there is no getting away from it, not even for a second. You can pretend to be happy, you can even convince yourself, momentarily, that life is good and all is well. But people know the truth. All they have to do is take one look at you; your body screams of the agony you face each and every day. There is no escape.

The other thing that makes me remember this day is one of the real reasons I wrote this book. "You'll lose weight when you're ready." Isn't that what we always hear? "When you've finally had enough, you'll be able to fix it." "When you hit rock bottom, you'll fight your way back up." "Trust me, you're a-ha moment will arrive and you'll know what to do."

But what if your "a-ha moment" never comes?

What if while waiting for lightning to strike, you give yourself a heart attack or a stroke, and you die?

Will that be your rock-bottom moment, once you're dead?

When I weighed 336 pounds, I was desperate to do anything to stop the vicious cycle I was on, anything to save my life. But I couldn't do it. I had all the tools: I read all the books, and I knew what to eat and what exercise I needed to do. I set out each day with a new plan for how I was going to beat this problem, once and for all.

But I always failed miserably. Self-doubt would creep in, no matter how hard I tried to beat it back. Temptation would take over my will, and I would find myself eating, and I couldn't stop. I consciously knew that my actions were going to cause my death, and yet I couldn't force myself to abstain. I was slowly killing myself with food, and I knew it.

The lady in the store seemed to think I wasn't ready to lose weight. Oh, really? Let's see. Just a year before, I'd given birth to a twelve-pound, seven-ounce baby because I'd been unable to get my gestational diabetes under control. It seems drinking a two-liter bottle of Mountain Dew every day isn't really good for one's blood sugar. Did I want to cause my unborn baby harm? Of course not. Did I want to die and leave my two young children without a mother? Desperately, no! I cried and I prayed and I begged God to please give me the strength, to please show me the way. Over the years I sought help from medical doctors, advice from therapists. Sometimes they brought a little success. Most of the time I was left with more failed attempts and broken promises to myself. Was I ready to lose weight and finally put the misery behind me? HELL, YES! But that didn't mean it happened. For sixteen years, it didn't happen. I grew fatter, my health deteriorated, and my already low self-esteem careened into oblivion. I felt so worthless, so helpless.

I surmised over the years that I was the problem. I was lazy. I didn't have discipline, self-control. I was weak. How else could I explain my inability to do something about my weight, to change my circumstances, to save my life? I blamed myself, and that certainly didn't help me solve the problem. It only heaped on more self-hatred, and I was collapsing underneath the weight of it all. Miserable doesn't even come close to describing how I felt.

I wrote *Designated Fat Girl* for those out there who are battling the same thing, who feel so trapped in this vicious, self-destructive cycle. I want you to know you are not alone and you are not crazy. Sometimes you can't solve the problem yourself and you need some help. And that's okay. Saving your sanity and your life is so much more important than saving face.

I also wrote this book so that others may somehow begin to understand that most obese people are not fat because they love food too much or because they are lazy and undisciplined. Many are addicted to food, just like an alcoholic who can't stop drinking, even if it is ruining their lives. I honestly feel as though our society does not recognize food addiction as a legitimate, serious condition. I am here to tell them, through my story, how very real and devastating it is. My hope is that others will see that it is not about the food.

My journey with morbid obesity spanned sixteen years; but I can't remember a time in which food was not an issue. I was a fat child and a chubby teenager. In high school I lost weight and convinced myself that yes, I could pursue my dream of being a broadcast journalist. I went away to college, met the man of my dreams, and landed a job on TV. My life was almost too perfect.

That's when the weight started to pile on. Within a year of getting married, I weighed 200 pounds. I quit my TV job because I thought the station would fire me for being too fat. The next ten years were filled with broken dreams: I couldn't pursue the career I wanted, and I felt too heavy to have the children my husband and I desperately desired. Eventually we did have two beautiful children, but the joy in watching them grow was about the only happiness I could find. I was depressed, I was hurt, and because I couldn't stop abusing food, I believe I was suicidal. I knew that my health was hanging on by a string, and I still was unable to help myself. I was going to die if I didn't do something. And finally I took action.

Some of this is hard for me to write. A lot of it may be difficult to read. But I vowed at the beginning of this process that I would be honest, no matter how uncomfortable. My hope is that someone hanging on the edge like I was will read this and feel hopeful. And that those who have loved ones who suffer from food addiction will gain some insight into this hideous disease. Sharing my story has been very helpful to my healing process; if it helps others as well, then my success is that much sweeter.

Death Via Drive-Thru

JUNE 2002

I just don't have the fight in me anymore. I've been battling myself for two solid days, part of a several-years-long war, and I am done. It's exhausting, and I simply don't have the strength. I am weak. I am a failure. I am a disgusting pig of a woman, and I'm tired of trying desperately to convince myself otherwise. What's the point? Ultimately I will lose. Sooner or later I will give in to the compulsion that has plagued me for almost a decade. Why not get it over with now? Save myself the added failure of this doomed charade. Go ahead and prove my subconscious right—the voice that started as a whisper when we arrived at the beach on Sunday—the same voice that now, on Tuesday, is a pitch above shrieking. YOU ARE A WORTH-LESS PIECE OF SHIT! YOU CAN'T CONTROL YOUR-SELF AND EVERYBODY KNOWS IT! THE LEAST YOU COULD DO IS HAVE THE GUTS TO ADMIT YOU NEED IT! YOU CAN'T LIVE WITHOUT IT! YOU WILL DIE WITHOUT IT! YOU ARE A SPINELESS WIMP!

The room is almost completely dark. The shades are drawn on the two tiny windows, but I can still see the smallest sliver of light blue sky, readying to make its retreat for the night. I've been in here for a long time, and I need to pee. But in here is safe and out there is a land mine of emotions that I don't want to face. Disappointment. Hurt. Disgust. I see it in their eyes when they look at me, or rather, when they glance at me for a millisecond before averting their gaze. It hurts to look at me. I avoid it as much as possible myself.

It suddenly occurs to me what a ridiculous pose I strike. Michael and I were both flabbergasted when we got stuck with the bedroom with twin beds. The other rooms in the rented bungalow were needed for various reasons by other family members, and so this was it. We'd discussed pushing the beds together; but after two nights, that has yet to happen. And here I lay, with my mounds of flesh hanging off both sides of my assigned cot. Not even the almost complete darkness nor my dark top and even darker pants can keep me from reaching a surprising realization: I no longer fit on a twin bed. After some ten years as an active member of the morbidly obese, I thought I'd identified and experienced every humiliation possible. If only that were really true.

I wonder how long I can hide out in here. Every time Michael comes to check on me—at last count, three—I feign sleep. It's a family vacation, and I am supposed to be spending time with family; instead I am in a dark room on a twin bed fighting with myself over whether or not I should eat. Sooner or later I'm going to have to go out and show myself. I will have to face my husband, who so doesn't deserve this, but whom I can't seem to treat the way he should be treated. He shows me nothing but love, care, and respect; in return he gets nothing but lies and a big fat mess of a wife. I often think I will burn in hell for the way I abuse the body that God gave me, but deep down I know it's my poor treatment of such a wonderful man that will haunt me for eternity.

I try to heave myself off the bed, but my middle is so large that it takes a few tries. My joints ache from lying there so long, and my head hurts from the tears that stain the pillow. I know what I must do, and my heart is heavy. I have to lie, again, and I have to go eat. There's no turning back now. The decision has been made and that's that. Time to get on with it already.

I turn on the light and immediately wince from the bare bright bulb hanging from the ceiling fan. As my eyes adjust, I go over to the small dresser that sits against the wall across from the beds. Grabbing a tissue, I blot at the black smears under my hazel eyes. I smooth down the wild, thin brown hair sticking up on my head. I press my clothes with both hands, willing the wrinkles to fall away. I shrug, knowing it really doesn't matter anyway. I look like a big piece of shit, and nothing I do in the next thirty seconds, thirty days, or thirty years is going to change that. Nothing.

I'm almost out the door before the plaintive wail from deep within me can finally be heard. *Don't do this! You've had two great days! Keep going! You are strong! You deserve better!*

My hand pauses in midair above the doorknob. I want to hear the other side of the argument; I long to believe that I am worth saving, that my life has meaning and value. But I've been caught in the middle of this psychological push-pull for most of my adult life, and the truth is, it's easier to believe the bad stuff. When you grow up assuming that you are worthless, it is an uphill battle even to try to think differently. Some days, like the last two, I am able to convince myself that yes, I am worthy.

Yes, I deserve happiness. I eat relatively well. I am able to beat back the voices of negativity that infest my psyche. But eventually the tide of self-hatred washes ashore, and it pulls with it every good intention of mine. I am breathless from the swift movement of all my hard work out to sea, and I am left drained and empty. I have no fight. I feel hopeless and doomed. I curl into a ball and let the ocean of misery reclaim my miserable soul. The final resignation, after hours and hours of going back and forth within myself, is a relief.

So it's decided, but it doesn't make the lie any easier. My heart pounding, I open the door and quickly step out into the hallway, before I change my mind yet again. All the other bedrooms in the house are dark; it appears everyone is either in the living room or the kitchen.

I slowly walk down the hall, making out the familiar sounds of the Madden NFL video game. Michael was like a kid, so excited to bring his Xbox so that he could play with his brother, Eddie. He had been looking forward to this vacation, so ready to spend time at the beach with his parents, his brother, his sister, and their families. I suppose he was happy to have me here, too, although I can't imagine why. Surely no one thought a beach trip would be a good thing for me. Fat girls and the beach go together like vegetarians and pig pickin's.

I reach the living room. Michael's video game is emblazoned on the too-large television teetering on the too-small television stand. He and Eddie are gesturing wildly with their controls, deeply enthralled in their play. They don't see me, their backs are to me, and I'm guessing not much could make them unglue their eyes from the screen. But little Eddie sees me. My three-month-old nephew is lying on a blanket on the floor, his little legs kicking wildly inside his sleeper, all fuzzy and blue and covered with little white lambs. He gives me a huge gummy grin, kicks harder, and flails his little arms with glee. My throat catches, as it has many times during this trip. *I want one of those,* I say to myself for the thousandth time. *Then don't do this,* that little voice finds another way to break the surface and get through to my conscious mind. But it's a futile effort. My fate—at least for this night—has already been decided.

"Touchdown!" Michael jumps up and pumps his fist into the air, while Eddie drops his face into his hands. It's obvious who is having the better game.

My stomach is fluttering with nerves, but I decide now is as good a time as any. "Hey." I try to sound casual, but I'm sure they'll see right through me. I swallow hard, waiting for their reaction to seeing me after all my time locked in my room.

It's anticlimactic, to say the least. "Hey, honey," Michael says, not looking up. He immediately laughs at Eddie. "How many times are you going to run that play, man? Give it up!"

I'm left standing there, stupidly. That's it? No questions, no looking me over? I'm dumbfounded . . . and a little ticked.

"I'm going to go out and get a newspaper," I say, waiting, almost willing Michael to whip around at me suspiciously, hitting me with questions. *Why do you need a newspaper? It's raining out. Should you be driving? Can I go with you?*

But there's none of that. "Okay," Michael says, and Eddie suddenly jumps up, as if doing so will improve his game. "Dude, where's my kicker?!"

And that's that. They're playing, and I'm standing behind the couch, fingering the little tassels hanging from an afghan thrown over the top. And I'm pissed. Predictably, I'm looking for someone to blame, and Michael has walked right into my trap. *How could you let me do this?* I silently scream at him. *Don't you see what I'm up to? Don't you care?*

Without another word, I grab my purse and my keys off the entryway table and walk out the door. Hot tears sting my eyes, but I'm not really sure why I'm crying now.

Do I really blame Michael for this? I know that can't possibly be true, but I am weary from the self-hatred in which I've wallowed all afternoon. I'm looking for a reprieve, if even for a little while. I brush the ill-conceived animosity toward Michael aside and get into my car.

We've only been at the beach for two days and I haven't driven by myself yet. With my horrible sense of direction, I just know I will get lost. Still, that doesn't stop me. I am pretty sure I can get to the grocery store, and what I am looking for won't be too far from that. I pull out of the main drive of the vacation resort and onto the highway. I breathe a deep sigh of relief. Finally I begin to let myself off the hook.

I turn on the radio. I hum a little with the familiar tune. The deal-making starts. *I've been really good the last two days,* I tell myself. *I've earned a little reward. I am on vacation, for Pete's sake. And, I'm here with my in-laws! Talk about stress! It's okay to go ahead and eat tonight. Tomorrow I can start fresh. Tomorrow there are five days left of this trip. Five solid days of eating right and exercising, and I can go home feeling good. Yes, a little treat tonight is in order. It'll help keep me motivated for the rest of my time here!*

Of course my reasoning is ridiculous. Of course my mood over the last several hours can only be described as manic. Beat myself up. Feel sorry for myself. Blame others. Pick myself up with lies. I know it's a twisted existence, but having that knowledge doesn't stop me from doing it, from living it. I've lived this way so long, I feel powerless to change it. I wouldn't even know where to start.

No, I'm not going to let the reality of my psychosis get me down now. This is one of the only happy times I get in a day, the period right before I eat. I've suffered the hours of indecision, and I have finally relented to the temptation. Now I can enjoy it, revel in it. There will be plenty of time later for more self-loathing, for sure.

I exit the highway, heading toward the bright fluorescent glow of the shopping center. I quickly find what I've been looking for, and I pull the car into the familiar drive-thru. No, I haven't been to this particular McDonald's before, but it doesn't matter. McDonald's is my home. My comfort. The people here have exactly what I need, and nothing is going to stop me from getting it.

I smile for the first time in two days.

"Welcome to McDonald's. May I take your order?" the voice crackles on the other end of the speaker. Sometimes the voice is friendly and inviting; sometimes it's rushed and annoyed. I suppose it doesn't really matter, as long as it is here to help me.

"Yes, I'd like a double cheeseburger meal, super-sized, with a Coke," I answer, not needing a menu. My order is always the same.

"Will that complete your order?"

No, it wouldn't. "Oh, I forgot. I also need a ten-piece Chicken McNugget Meal with a Sprite, please." I don't know why I feel the need to try and make it sound like I'm ordering for two people, feigning forgetfulness and ordering a different drink with the second meal. Do I really care what the lady at McDonald's thinks of me?

"Is that super-sized, too?" the disembodied voice asks.

"No thanks," I say cheerily. No need to act like a pig. I crack myself up.

"Pull up to the window for your total."

As I wait for my food, I wonder, bemusedly, how much money I've spent on fast food in my lifetime. Surely it is in the thousands of dollars. I feel a twinge of guilt, but I quickly stuff it down, turning up the radio and singing along. I refuse to feel bad now. In my mind the drive-thru line is my safe zone.

The smell of salt and grease fills me with joy. My mouth waters, and my throat aches for those first tastes. It's been two whole days, an amazing amount of restraint on my part. My pulse quickens as the car in front of me pulls off and I move forward. I pay the lady and ask for extra ketchup. She gives me my change and my food and drinks. I haven't even pulled away from the window before I am reaching into the bag for a handful of fries. I stuff them into my mouth, wincing from the heat, but chewing heartily anyway. They burn a little, but I don't care. Now, for a brief moment, I don't feel quite so empty.

I have almost finished the first carton of fries before I pull into the parking space in front of the grocery store. I suppose the rain is keeping folks inside, as there are few cars in the parking lot. I don't feel self-conscious at all as I polish off the double cheeseburger in record time. The ache in my stomach is beginning to dissipate, but I still want more. My mind is blank as I finish off the second batch of fries. I finally stop eating long enough to take a long slurp of Coke, enjoying the burn of the carbonation on my throat. I dust off the salt on my fingers and wipe the grease off my hands with a napkin. I take the box of chicken nuggets out of the bag and replace it with the trash from my eaten food. I take the bag and the Sprite and get out of the car. It's a dance I've danced many, many times, and I have the moves down to a science. I throw the trash and the untouched soda in a wastebasket in front of the store and walk inside.

I wonder if I smell like fried food. *Better get something for the car,* I tell myself, making my way down the refrigerated section first. I start to grab an individual carton of Häagen-Dazs, but I think better of it and instead get a gallon of Breyers Chocolate Ripple. I then pick up a can of air freshener and a newspaper. As I wait in line to pay for my items, I grab a Hershey's chocolate bar and a package of Reese's Peanut Butter Cups. I pay without making eye contact with the cashier. Suddenly worried about the time, I hurry back to the car.

The parking lot is still pretty empty. I down the ten chicken nuggets in about two minutes flat. I gulp the rest of the Coke. I pull out of the parking lot. Despite the rain, I roll down all the windows on the car, letting the air circulate, hoping to rid the car of the greasy smell of my transgressions. Making sure there are no witnesses, I throw the chicken nuggets box and the soda cup out the window before turning back onto the highway.

I feel nothing. I'm full, at least for the moment, so there's no need to belittle myself or try to make myself feel better. Despite the large volume of food I ate in such a small amount of time, I don't feel sick. That is a blessing. It allows me, if only briefly, to feel satisfied. These short periods don't come often, and I allow myself to listen to the wind cleansing the inside of my car and my mind. My thoughts are turned down, and I am somewhat at peace.

In no time I am back in front of our bungalow. No sign that Michael is looking for me. I wonder if he even really noticed I left. I should feel relieved, but I'm not. The tiniest amount of regret starts to seep in, but I push it down by lashing out at my husband. *How could he let me down this way? How will I ever get better if he can't be bothered to pay attention?* I feel the rush of emotions start to rise up, but then I remember the candy and the ice cream. The anger and resentment, the guilt and the remorse, fade away quickly. I spray the inside of the car with the air freshener before rolling the windows back up. Once out of the car, I spray my clothes ever so slightly, hoping to disguise where I've been and what I've been up to. I put the can deep inside my trunk. I take the candy bars out of the bag and put them inside my purse. I head inside with the grocery bag and the newspaper.

Michael and Eddie are still playing the game, but this time Michael looks up at me as I walk in. "Hey, I was worried about you," he says, coming over to me. I hope he can't smell anything.

I can see the worry in his eyes, and I feel that familiar pang. At this point I've felt it so much, it's as familiar to me as any other emotion. "Sorry, I got a little lost." I lie, knowing he will believe it, and feel all the more guilty.

"What's in the bag?" he asks.

"Oh, I got us some ice cream," I say, perhaps a little too brightly.

"Did someone say ice cream?" Eddie's wife, Molly, comes in from the other room, holding the baby. He's asleep on her shoulder.

Molly. Thank goodness she's so nice, or I swear I'd have to kill her. She's a size 4, soaking wet, and she's given her husband two children. For those keeping score, that's one thing I'll never be (a size 4), and one thing I'm starting to think I'll never be able to do (give my husband children).

I hand the bag to Molly, and she takes it into the kitchen. I put down my purse and keys on the entry table. I'm still holding the newspaper. I meet Michael's eyes.

"Ice cream?" he asks softly. It's not an accusation, and I don't take it as one. I feel too guilty to be defensive.

"Yeah," I say casually. "I've been good all day, and I figured a little bit won't hurt. We *are* on vacation, you know," I say with a little smile.

He smiles back. "You have been good today." He pulls me close to him and hugs me firmly, protectively. I feel as though I will jump out of my skin. I love him so very much, but I can't stand to be touched. It makes my skin crawl. All I can think of is how my body must feel under his arms, and I am repulsed for him. I force myself to hug him back, and I feel the sting of salt again, but this time it's not on my lips, but in my eyes.

We join Eddie and Molly in the kitchen, where I have a
very conservative bowl of ice cream. There's talk of asking
Michael's parents and the other family members to join us, but
there's no answer when Eddie tries to call their cottage. Thank
God. I know what's going to happen to me emotionally once
I am alone again, and I don't need a whopping dose of in-law
inadequacy on top of it. I don't think I could take it.

Michael and Eddie return to their video game, and Molly
goes to put the baby down. I excuse myself to the restroom. My
stomach is now starting to pay the price of the sins of the past
hour, and I'm in the bathroom for a while. This is where the
guilt really starts. I lied to Michael's face, although that really
was nothing new. He was concerned about me, and I'd spent
much of the evening blaming him for something I knew good
and well was all my fault. I'd taken the last two days of eating
reasonably well and thrown them away as if they meant nothing. *But I'm going to start fresh tomorrow,* the little voice inside
says, rather weakly. Tomorrow. Always tomorrow.

After I clean up, I look at the full-length mirror on the back
of the bathroom door. I wish I could say the reflection of my
almost three-hundred-pound frame is a shock, but it isn't. I am
long used to the grotesque figure I've become. My face is so
swollen, it's hard to recognize the person I was just a few short
years ago. My skin is dry and scaly, my hair is lifeless and limp.
And my stomach . . . I can't look at it for more than a few seconds without forcing myself to look away, like a bright light that
burns your eyes and leaves you seeing spots for hours. I look in
the mirror and I see a monster—a hideous beast that has taken
over my body and my life. I am too weak to fight him off. He has

control, and I am powerless to do anything about it. Eventually, I am sure, the beast will kill me.

I go back to our room and quietly shut the door. I should go out and say goodnight to everyone, but I am too ashamed. I just want to go to sleep, to not hurt, if just for a few hours. I am never overweight in my dreams; I am thin and young and pretty. Self-hatred is nowhere to be found, and I retreat to that place whenever I can. It is my one escape, my chance to get out from under the death grip I feel most of the time.

I change quickly, although it occurs to me the ritual is pretty silly. I take off my drab T-shirt and pants and put on a drabber T-shirt and shorts. No pretty lingerie, no cute cotton pajamas for me. As it is I'd die if anyone saw my bare legs in the shorts I wear to bed; I haven't worn shorts or skirts in public for years.

I turn out the lights and lie in bed, begging for sleep to come, but it eludes me. As silent tears slide down my face, I feel as though the grief will overtake me. *Please God,* I pray to myself. *Please help me. I don't know how to stop this. I can't do it alone. I need help. I feel like I'm going to die.*

My cries no longer want to be muted, and I roll over so that I can sob into my pillow. I think of how much time has been lost, how much of our lives have been ruined by this hideous disease. I think about the future, and I cry even harder. What could the coming years possibly hold for us? Children are out of the question; my doctor doubted I could even get pregnant. I'm too heavy. And even if I could conceive, the pregnancy would be too dangerous for me and for the baby. Wouldn't my in-laws just love that? No, there are no kids in our future, not if I can't get this problem under control. And I see no sign of my getting a grip, despite the promises I made myself earlier. For the first time all night, I am being honest with myself. I am in a very sick place, and I know it. But I don't know how to fix it. Really fix it, I mean. Not with deal making or grandiose, unrealistic plans. How can I finally fix *me?*

The tears let up. I get up to grab some tissue, maneuvering in the dark room over to the dresser. My purse on the floor catches my eye. Michael must have put it in here while I was in the bathroom. I wipe my face and blow my nose, suddenly remembering what's inside my pocketbook. My pulse quickens a little. I grab my purse and climb back into bed. *I can get up early in the morning, before anyone else. I can walk on the beach, down to the pier and back. That's got to be a couple of miles, right? Yes. Yes, I can do that in the morning, and then maybe I can do it in the evening, too. You know, really make a strong effort. Michael's parents are bound to notice that. And Michael, too . . . he will be so proud of me.* I sniff away the tears as I open my purse and dig out the chocolate. *And because I'm walking first thing in the morning, I will set the tone for the rest of the day. I will eat well because I won't want to mess up what I've done.* I rip open the Hershey's bar. *But maybe you should start now. You don't need that candy. Throw it away. Prove to yourself that you know you are worth it.* The little voice is annoying me now, and I push it deep inside my subconscious. *No, I have to eat this now,* I tell myself. *If I don't, I'll feel deprived all day tomorrow, and that will mess me up. Go ahead and get it over with and then make a fresh start.*

I lie in bed and eat the Hershey's bar, and then the Reese's cups. I stuff the wrappers between the two mattresses, vowing to get rid of them the next morning. My tears are long gone. I'm back to feeling nothing. The back-and-forth has stopped, at least for now, and I'm ready to let sleep come and get me. Take me away. Take me to thin, pretty, happy Jennifer. I miss her. So much.

I fall asleep.

The beast smiles.

2

Bingeing and Hiding

My binge eating was born in 1990. I was a senior in high school, and I had just gone through yet another breakup with my abusive boyfriend. I decided the answer to all my problems would be to finally rid myself of the extra thirty pounds I'd carried for as long as I could remember. I wish I could say I wanted to lose the weight to attract a better boyfriend, but in truth, I hoped to make the abusive one insanely jealous so he would fall head over heels for me and never cheat again. Twisted, I know, but that's where my head was that New Year's Eve. I decided to stay home and eat all my favorite foods, to get them out of my system. Then the next day I would start my new diet in earnest. I got a double cheeseburger and fries from Wendy's, plus a big bag of Funyuns and a two-liter bottle of Mountain Dew. I stayed home and watched Dick Clark and ate until I thought I would puke. This was new; it had never occurred to me before to binge like this. Looking back, I have no clue what gave me the idea.

At midnight the Wendy's meal was long gone. I threw away what was left of the Funyuns, and I poured the remaining Mountain Dew down the sink. I was so satisfied with myself.

Believe it or not, it worked. I lost twenty-five pounds in about three months. I taught myself to drink diet soft drinks, something I never thought I would do.

I avoided fast food and Funyuns, and I even started to exercise a little. I received compliments everywhere I went. The more attention I got, the more motivated I became to keep up the good work.

The abusive boyfriend was jealous, and he wanted me back. Of course I went. And I did keep the weight off for quite some time, so I became convinced that bingeing was the way to go. Get it out of your system; then get down to work.

Little did I know that this dangerous bingeing habit would one day threaten my life.

I can't remember a time when eating wasn't a central part of my being. I wasn't an obese child, but in some ways I think I had it even worse: I was always about twenty-five pounds overweight, just fat enough to get picked on. Where did the extra weight come from? Genetics, I'm sure played a part, although neither of my parents was overweight. Smoking was their vice of choice, with the added inclination of drinking for my dad. I have two brothers, one of whom was skinny as a rail and short most of his life. The other, like me, has always fought extra pounds, despite his being a highly decorated athlete while growing up. No, my extra weight was born more out of poor habits, caring way too much way too early about the wrong kinds of food. Fast food wasn't the problem then; a trip to McDonald's was a rare treat when I was a little girl. But soda— or "drinks" as we used to call them in North Carolina—that was my problem almost from the very beginning.

My love affair with Mountain Dew goes back as far as I can remember. My dad would get home from his job at the carton factory in the early afternoon, right after we got home from school. He would send one of us down to the corner store to buy our daily snack. We each got to choose something to eat and something to drink. We also had to get something for Dad. My brothers and my father always varied their choices. Sometimes my dad would get these pink cupcakes called "snowballs"; other times, he'd want a long package of peanuts and a Pepsi. My brothers liked all kinds of chips and cakes and cookies. But my choice was always the same: a bag of Funyuns and a Mountain Dew. There was nothing better than that salty-sweet mix, and it was part of my afternoon routine for years and years.

I can remember my mom going to the grocery store every Saturday and coming home with a large bag of potato chips, a box of Ho Hos, and a two-liter bottle of Pepsi. Those snacks would be gone by the afternoon, my brothers and I hurrying to eat them before they disappeared. There was always a definite competition in my house for food.

I smile now when I think about how much I complain about my kids being picky eaters, because really, they are nothing compared to my brothers and me. I would eat no fruit whatsoever. I couldn't stand the texture of it, and to this day I don't eat any. I would eat very few vegetables, either. Sometimes my mom could get us to eat green beans with fatback or corn on the cob smothered in butter. I never wanted to try new things; I always hated going over to other people's houses to eat. I can remember having lunch at my friend Michelle's house. I was probably five years old. Her mother put the plate in front of me, and I stared at the brown bread. Brown bread? I'd never seen such a thing. And I wasn't about to put it in my mouth. I was too ashamed to come out and say it, so I did what any five-year-old would do. I waited until Michelle's mother wasn't looking and I threw the bread on the floor, under the table. Problem solved.

Michelle's parents were professors at Duke University and were obviously a little more enlightened when it came to healthy eating. I remember bringing over a bag of Funyuns to share with Michelle, and her father asked to see the bag. He turned it over and began reading the ingredients. I couldn't imagine what he was doing, and I don't remember his ultimate verdict.

No, my parents were not college professors. We were a distinctly blue-collar family with enough money to get by but not a whole lot left over. Food was a cheap way to show love and bring pleasure. Not only did my dad buy us afternoon snacks, but he also would make mammoth "Daddy Burgers" on the grill, each thick patty smothered with mounds of cheese. My mom would cook her own french fries in our FryDaddy. And sweet tea flowed freely. Whenever we had a hankerin' for dessert, my brothers and I knew to look in Dad's top dresser drawer—he always had cookies or candy bars stashed there. When we were out of school for the summer, Mom would leave us a dollar each to go to the store and buy whatever we wanted to eat. My brothers and I fought like cats and dogs, but I can distinctly remember my brother Jimmy and I pooling our money once and buying a Chef Boyardee Pizza Kit. Making that pizza with Jimmy is something I remember fondly.

Every memory, every special occasion, was tied up with food—and still is. My first thought when I wake up in the morning is, *What will I eat today?* My last thought when I go to sleep is, *What will I eat tomorrow?* If I know a special occasion is coming up, I ponder all the food possibilities. It occupies my every waking thought.

College brought a whole new level of food independence. I was still twenty-five pounds lighter, and I managed to keep most of it off freshman year. But it occurred to me that I could have anything I wanted to eat, anytime I wanted. No longer was I limited to the one soft drink a day Dad bought for an afternoon snack; the campus cafeteria had all the soda I could want, on tap. I brought a refrigerator to school, and my room-mate provided a microwave. This brought all new possibilities: I could eat sugarcoated cereal for breakfast every morning, and microwave pizza in our room. Probably the most damaging part of my newfound food freedom was burger baskets. I was stuck on campus without a car, and back then there were no fast-food places in our little college town. But we had an on-campus burger joint, and I made a regular practice of order-ing a hamburger-and-fries basket. I remember being in awe of the fact that I could do this at 9:00 and 10:00 p.m., long after I'd eaten dinner. *I can do this to get through my studying,* I told myself. *I just need a pick-me-up.* How I didn't gain all my weight back and more that freshman year, I'll never know. But it would happen soon enough.

By my sophomore year I was living off campus with a roommate. I was also commuting an hour and a half each way to work as a reporter at a television station in South Carolina. I worked horrible hours and had to drive miles and miles on the interstate. This was where my fast-food addiction really heated up. I was working late. I was tired. I was stressed from the job, the commute, the full load of courses I was taking and, oh yeah, I was planning a wedding. It was almost too easy to give in to the temptation of the many fast-food places up and down I-95, most of which were open twenty-four hours. I found myself stopping for burgers and fries at midnight three and four times a week, always telling myself that this was the last time, I just needed it to get through the commute. Famous last words.

I definitely was eating more fast food, but I wasn't at the bingeing point yet. That would come just a little later, when the weight started to pile on from the extra burgers and fries and endless soda. The stress from gaining weight and all the other things in my life started to get to me, and in a desperate attempt to stop the madness, I would employ what worked so well for me on that New Year's Eve back in 1990. I would load up on fast food, promising myself that this was the last time, all I needed was to get it out of my system. But more and more I found that what I thought was a foolproof method no longer worked. My resolve would erode quickly, and I would eat more. The weight began to pile on even more, and for the first time in my life, I entered a weight class I never thought I would achieve. The more I tried to fix it, the worse it became. I felt as though I was sinking in quicksand.

Over the years, I brought bingeing to an art form. It usually centered around fast food, but not always. Sometimes I couldn't leave the house, afraid Michael would know what I was up to. I would take a loaf of bread, a jar of pasta sauce, and a tub of butter, and over the course of an afternoon, I would eat all of it. I would tell Michael I was "working" in our second bedroom that I used as an office. And I would just eat and eat and eat. I eventually would get sick and have to go to the bathroom, but if I waited just a little while, I was ready to eat again. And again and again.

Fast food was always my drug of choice, though. In early 2000 I started a new job that had me commuting an hour each way, again along the interstate. I would call Pizza Hut before I left work for the day. Imagine how mortified I was when they knew me by my order, "Ms. Joyner? Oh yes, a medium pepperoni and sausage pizza and a twenty-ounce Mountain Dew?" I sheepishly said, "Yes," and left to pick up my food. I was embarrassed to be remembered for my standing order, especially when the purchase of a single drink must have clued the folks into the fact that this was indeed a meal for one. But not too embarrassed to keep going.

I could down the whole pizza in the first twenty minutes or so of my hour-long drive home. Then, when I was halfway there, I would stop off the interstate and hit McDonald's for a double cheeseburger meal. By the time I finished that, I was home and felt pretty sick. But I'd go to the bathroom and wait a few minutes, and then I was ready to go again. Sometimes I would have a full dinner with Michael.

Other times I'd go to the grocery store and get a pint of Häagen-Dazs and eat it in my office, telling Michael again that I was working. Sometimes I would forget to throw the trash away from my binge eating, and I would see that Michael had found it in my car and thrown it away himself.

I was so ashamed, but I felt powerless to stop it. Michael would complain that my car smelled like ketchup. If we rode together on the weekends, he would sigh heavily and roll the windows down, unable to take the smell. I said nothing. What could I say? Promise not to do it again? Even I, in my advanced stage of denial, knew those promises were empty.

After a day of binge eating, I would have what I call a "binge hangover" the next morning. I would feel so gassy, so bloated. My stomach would ache, and I would have to go to the bathroom several times. I would have no energy, and worse, I had incredible guilt and remorse.

I suppose that's why I would hardly ever binge in the mornings; that was a time for regret and repurpose. I would set out each day to right the wrongs of the day before. If I was lucky, I could make it for a couple of days without bingeing again. At my worst my resolve was gone by lunchtime.

There was such shame surrounding what I was doing to myself and to my body that I kept it hidden as much as I could. Still, someone who is addicted to food isn't allowed the luxury of anonymity; we wear our failures on our bodies for the world to see. I used to be envious of people with drug or alcohol problems. At least they could hide their addictions, if even for a little while, from the rest of the population. A fat person might as well wear a sign with flashing neon lights: I CAN'T CONTROL MYSELF!

Indeed eating in public is a no-win situation for the obese. If we eat a lot, people stare and confirm for themselves what they'd already been thinking. If we eat a little, people smirk, knowing full well there's more to the story. Thus I did whatever I had to do to avoid eating in public. At work I would eat lunch in my car, away from prying eyes. At family gatherings I would put the bare minimum on my plate. I suppose this is the behavior that prompted my father-in-law to once ask me if I hid food. It was pretty early in our marriage, and I'm sure Michael's parents were struggling for answers as they saw me spiral out of control. When I tearfully confessed to them that I was trying to get my weight under control, Mr. Joyner said he knew a man who would find candy wrappers stuffed into desk drawers at his home, knowing that they belonged to his wife. Was that what I was doing? I told him yes, although I really, at that point, didn't hide food at home. Perhaps that's where I got the idea to do so, because I did actually do that many years later. You would think the humiliation I endured as the result of my father-in-law's questions would shame me into finally doing something about my eating. You would think.

The bingeing and the hiding of food made me feel even lonelier. Being a fat woman is one of the loneliest things you can be. Family and friends want to help you, but they don't know how, and they're afraid to say the wrong thing, so they usually don't say anything. I've found that when I have tried to bring it up, even with Michael, it makes others very uncomfortable, and I usually just drop the subject. Fat women don't even acknowledge other fat women, because doing so means you are one of them, and most of us want to deny that as long as possible. You can't even commiserate with those who understand best. So you keep everything inside, struggling and hurting all alone.

It didn't help that a great deal of my eating was in the car, either commuting to and from work or—worse—sneaking out of the house to eat, telling Michael I was going to the store or running some other errand. Mealtimes for fat people are not the social gatherings that others enjoy. Instead they are desperate times filled with self-hatred and broken promises. When the eating is finished, the deal making begins. And on and on it goes.

Sometimes I wonder how many cheeseburgers I've had in my lifetime, how many french fries I have eaten. How much space would all of my trash take up at the landfill? I swear, with all the meals I have purchased, I wonder, how could I have never won one of those fast-food giveaways? You know, like the Monopoly games at McDonald's? Certainly my odds at winning were better than most. But alas, I have not won anything from eating fast food.

When it became vogue to sue fast-food chains for various reasons, I had to chuckle. Were these people really serious? Yes, fast food had done a ton of damage to my health and to my happiness, but whose fault was that? Could I ever blame someone else for something I chose to do, even though I felt powerless to stop it? I think we all know that large quantities of fast food are harmful to the body, and we don't need movies like *Super Size Me* to prove it. I suppose eating fast food for our generation is like smoking was to our parents' generation. Smoking for my parents was the cool, cheap way to get your kicks. But now we know how harmful it is to the body, and our parents are hopelessly addicted. My generation has gotten used to fast food as a cheap and convenient way to eat, but we're starting to see how bad it is for our health. Hopefully it's a lesson we can help our kids learn early.

Now that I am a parent, I am so completely paranoid about what and how my kids eat. I really don't blame my parents for the way I turned out, yet I know that if I'd had a better idea of healthier eating habits from an earlier age, then perhaps the struggle wouldn't have been so mighty. In any case, I vowed not to let my kids eat crap. When my daughter, Emma, was just three months old, I caught my brother about to put his finger in her mouth, a finger that held the slightest dollop of whipped cream from a piece of apple pie. My mother was holding Emma and smiling broadly as Uncle Jimmy prepared to give her a treat. My screams caused Jimmy to jump back, and my mother almost dropped the baby. "WHAT ARE YOU DOING?" I shrieked, grabbing Emma in a huff. How dare they do something like that! Of course, they thought I was overreacting, but really, three months old? Yeah, I think that's a little early. Besides, couldn't they understand where I was coming from? I simply wanted to avoid future heartache for my child.

So I scrutinize everything that goes into my kids' mouths. But much to my chagrin, I have a couple of picky eaters to raise. On the one hand, both Emma and my son, Eli, will eat almost any kind of fruit. That makes my heart sing, especially since I don't touch the stuff. Vegetables are a different story. Emma will eat broccoli, but only with cheese. She'll eat green beans, begrudgingly. She'll eat green lettuce and cucumbers—and every once in a while, a raw carrot or two. But that's about it. And Eli, at four years old, won't let any vegetables come near him. Nothing. I bribe, I plead, I beg, but it's not happening. Still, they don't drink soda, and we limit fast food to the "rare" category. Emma will drink her weight in milk, and Eli likes apple juice a little too much, but at least they're doing much better than I ever did as a kid.

Eating has always been an issue for me, and I suppose it always will be. Again, I can't help but be a little jealous of a substance abuser. When a drug addict begins recovery, he can plan to avoid situations in which he's tempted to indulge. A food addict isn't so lucky. I have to eat in order to live. And temptation is everywhere.

3

I'm Jennifer Joyner, and I'm Not on TV

JANUARY 1994

If I'm really quiet, maybe no one will hear me. I listen as high heels click-clack on the tile floor, making their way to the stall on the far side of the television station's public bathroom. Whoever she is, she's fast. Just barely a minute, and she's already done her business, flushed, and is now washing her hands. I imagine her fixing her hair in the mirror as I hear the clang of bangles coming together. One of the anchors, no doubt. I pray that her primping will be brief, and mercifully, it is. The nameless, faceless woman click-clacks her way out the door, and once again I am alone, huddled down in a stall.

I'm ready for the tears to come—am willing them out of me—but curiously, nothing. I know the cry is there; the sorrow building in my chest threatens to cut off my very breath. I just want it out, I just want to release it, be free of it, make it finally happen so I can begin to let it go. But . . . nothing. Can't make myself cry. Can't feel the pain anymore. I'm numb.

I start to go over the events of the last hour, hoping the recollection will make the dam burst. I arrived at work a little before 5:00 p.m., ready for my evening shift as a reporter for WPDE-TV in Florence, South Carolina. It was only a part-time job, but I was just twenty-one years old, a junior in college. I wasn't even out of school yet, and I'd already landed an on-air television gig. Everyone told me that was unheard of, that my future was as bright as they come. Funny . . . there's nothing bright as I sit alone in a dingy bathroom trying to make myself sob.

My assignment this evening is to cover a PTA meeting at a local high school. It makes me chuckle when I think of how people think the life of a TV reporter is glamorous; I was going to spend my night in a school cafeteria, trying to get parents to talk to me about the rising rate of student violence. I was going to drive myself to the story (and I was horrible with directions), lug about forty pounds of camera equipment all alone, and shoot and edit the story myself, all on a 10:00 p.m. deadline. Glamorous? Hardly. Stressful? Unbelievably so, especially when you consider the current state of my affairs: I had just hit two hundred pounds. I was constantly paranoid that my bosses would fire me at any minute; after all, how many fat people do you see on TV? I felt their eyes on me as I walked around the newsroom, and I tried to brush it off, tried to feel better by reminding myself I had been good all week. I was limiting my calories, sticking to diet sodas, and watching my portion sizes. I had managed to walk a couple of miles at the campus track three times that week and had plans to do it again the next day. I hadn't yet stepped on the scale, but I was starting to feel somewhat confident in my efforts. Surely this would work! In no time I would lose the twenty pounds I'd gained since I started working there, and I would keep right on losing. My career would be set, and I would be so happy, finally so fulfilled. I keep telling myself that as I work, trying to avoid the prying eyes of the newsroom.

Because my meeting doesn't start until 7:00 p.m., my job is to help everyone prepare for the 6:00 p.m. newscast. Again, say good-bye to all the glamorous television news life theories—that prep work includes ripping apart scripts and sorting them into piles for the news and sports anchors, as well as for the director and producer of the show. I am also asked to run the teleprompter for the newscast—meaning I have to sit off to the side of the set and operate the conveyor belt that carries the words the anchors read on-screen. It is mind-numbing work, but I just chalk it up to paying my dues. I settle into the cold studio for what I expect will be an uneventful newscast.

Five minutes in the scurrying begins. Our weather anchor originated out of another studio hundreds of miles away in Myrtle Beach, but the feed for his shot is down. Everyone scrambles, trying to find a replacement, someone who can do the weather at the last minute, from our studio. "Go find Steve Hawley! He's done weather before!" One of the anchors calls out during a commercial break. A moment later Steve rushes into the studio, out of breath. "I didn't bring my jacket today!" He has a shirt and tie, but because he'd helped sports earlier, he doesn't have his blazer. We all look at each other helplessly as the floor manager ticks down how long we have until the commercial break is over. "Thirty seconds!"

Steve looks over at me, reluctantly. As he starts to walk over, I'm confused. How can I help? "Twenty seconds!"

Steve picks up the pace. "Jennifer!" he whispers, urgently. "I need your jacket!"

I don't have time to be embarrassed, humiliated. And I suppose I don't think to be right away. Time is of the essence, and I'm in a hurry to help any way I can. I jump up from the teleprompter station and take off my black blazer. It isn't until Steve throws it on, and not only does it fit, but it is a little loose, that the lump starts to form in my throat. Steve is not a small man; he is over six feet tall and has a nice masculine build. The fact that my jacket fits him makes my cheeks flush and my eyes smart instantly. Everyone in the studio looks away immediately, suddenly very busy with getting into place and shuffling papers. Steve makes it over to the weather wall just as the floor manager ticks down the final seconds with his hand. Crisis averted. The show goes on.

I sit at my teleprompter station, and, as discreetly as I can, untuck the purple shell out of my black skirt. No need to add to my humiliation by having the fat rolls once disguised by my jacket now on display. Tears threaten to spill over, but I can't allow it. What has happened is bad enough; I don't want to add to my humiliation at this point.

The weather segment ends, and Steve walks over to me, sheepishly. With as little fanfare as possible, he takes off the jacket and hands it over. "You're a lifesaver!" he says, a little too enthusiastically. I beam up at him, my smile equaling his banter. "No problem!" I reply. He quickly shuffles out, and I quickly put the coat back on as discreetly as I can.

The rest of the newscast is a blur. I bite my lip and focus on the teleprompter belt, pushing the tears as far down as I can. My face feels hot, and I can't look at anyone. When the final credits wrap, I bolt.

I already feel as though I could be fired at any minute because of how I look, and this certainly doesn't do anything to boost my confidence. I'm a rookie reporter with limited experience, and my weight is definitely an issue. How long can it be before they let me go? Every day I fear I will get called into the news director's office and given the boot. I'm incredibly anxious, and my anxiety drives me to eat. It's a vicious cycle.

☙❧

It was a miracle I was even in a newsroom in the first place. Growing up chubby and with low self-esteem, you wouldn't think I would conclude that broadcast journalism was the perfect career choice for me. Indeed I feared from the beginning my looks would be a sticking point, a fact that I would have to work around. But I'd always known since I was a little girl that I wanted to be a reporter. I can remember starting my own newspaper when I was nine years old, the *Neighborhood Observer*. I would ride around on my purple bike with the pink basket, gathering news stories about the Walkers' cat who was missing or the exchange student staying at the Davenport house. I'd type up the stories and deliver them to my neighbors, ringing the doorbell and running away in my shyness. As a freshman in high school, I became the representative of my high school for the Saturday page of the local newspaper—a real job that paid real money! News just fit with me, it felt natural.

Public speaking also came very naturally to me. I couldn't hold a tune, and acting wasn't my thing, so instead of singing or performing, I was always chosen to host school choir events or serve as narrator for school plays. In high school I got to make the announcements on the loudspeaker every afternoon, something that gave me such a rush. I really enjoyed being the one telling people what was going on.

Around my junior year of high school I put the two skills together and decided I should go after broadcast journalism. I knew I had reporting skills, and everyone told me I had a good voice. I also knew that my looks were average at best, and my weight was an issue. But back then it wasn't too hard to imagine that I could be on television. Not everyone looked like a Barbie doll, and I just figured my skills and hard work would make up for any physical shortcomings. I found a college with an excellent broadcast journalism department and I went for it.

As a freshman at the University of North Carolina at Pembroke, I shined. The school ran its own television station, and I immediately set my sights on being a news anchor. It was a small enough program that I got my audition pretty quickly. I tried out for weatherperson, and I nailed it. I was ecstatic when I got the job and thrilled that I was on my way to realizing my dream.

I have WPSU-TV to thank for my first real on-air job; I also have the television station to thank for introducing me to my future husband! Michael was a senior and a whiz at all things technical. I was miserably inept at running the equipment, and Michael took me under his wing and helped me out. I was head over heels in no time, and by the end of my freshman year, we were inseparable.

My sophomore year I heard about the Florence job and felt I had to try to get it. The pay was extremely low and the distance was great, but I knew it was an amazing opportunity, one that I had to at least give a shot. I was about 180 pounds at the time, my journey of real weight gain just beginning. I was ashamed of my appearance, but I didn't let it stop me. I bought the best size-16 suit I could find, and I got my hair professionally styled for my job interview. I went in and tried not to vomit from fear as the news director led me to his office. He was a very nice man, and we talked easily. He suggested I go up on the anchor desk and try reading from the teleprompter. An impromptu audition, if you will. I practiced deep breathing as I sat and waited for the lighting to be adjusted. Soon I was given a cue, and I read the script. It was a good audition. I felt great about my delivery, and I thought things were going pretty well.

The news director came out of the booth and joined me at the desk. "You are a natural," he said, and I beamed. My instincts were right; I was made for this kind of job! I was still shining when he leaned in to talk to me more quietly. "Can I give you some advice?" he asked. I nodded eagerly, waiting to soak in any and all information that would help me fulfill my dream. "You may want to try sitting at a slight angle," he said, still talking low so that the others in the crew couldn't hear him. I must have looked confused, because he went on to explain. "When I was a reporter, I was quite heavy," he started slowly. "When I was on the air, I learned to sit at an angle so I didn't look so broad to the viewer," he smiled warmly and patted my arm. I nodded and swallowed hard. I had hoped my looks, and especially my weight, wouldn't be a factor this early in the game. And I had thought the interview had gone so well. But clearly the news director was so distracted by my girth that he was forced to give me this advice. As he led me back into the newsroom, I steeled myself to receive the bad news: I wasn't going to get the job. I was simply too fat.

Surprisingly I was wrong. The news director offered me the job on the spot. I tried not to look too surprised as I happily accepted. I did it! I actually landed a real job at a real television station! Despite my looks! For a moment I was on cloud nine.

The moment didn't last very long. I was paranoid from the moment I started working there, surrounded by gorgeous, skinny twentysomethings who, like me, were hungry to get their careers started, but didn't face the physical challenges I did. My female coworkers wore cute tailored jackets and skirts; I struggled to find size-18 clothes that were suitable for me to wear on the air and didn't make me look as though I was wearing a circus tent. We all had to shoot our own stories, and it was physically taxing to lug around all the camera equipment. I would return to the station, huffing, puffing, and sweating from an evening of gathering news, hoping no one noticed my ill-fitting clothes or red, slick-with-perspiration face. One of the interns in the station told me that a reporter from a competing station had stopped him to ask about me, referring to me as "the healthy new reporter." I laughed it off, but boy did it sting, and I began to imagine that everyone was talking about the fat new girl, wondering how she'd landed the job. While my weight hadn't kept me from getting hired, I just knew that it would eventually cost me my job. And the more I worried, the more I ate . . . and the cycle continued. I just couldn't get a grip.

My dream was to be a television reporter. But the reality of the dream was like living a nightmare—it was physically difficult to do the job, and the mental toll of carrying around such anxiety was more than I could bear. Every day when I went to work, I expected to be called into the news director's office and be fired. I honestly felt I was just as good as any reporter there, but my issues with my appearance undermined my confidence at every turn. In the end, convinced it was the only way to save a shred of dignity, I quit. I'd only worked the job for thirteen months, and it broke my heart to give it up, especially under those circumstances. I just felt I had no other choice. I told my news director I needed to concentrate on finishing school and on my new marriage. I didn't mention my mounting weight, and thankfully, neither did he. He wished me well, and that was that. I left the job I had wanted more than anything.

I was sad to leave and ashamed that I was unable to get my weight under control and keep the job. But I honestly felt like it was a temporary setback; I never once, at that time, thought my television career was over. I just needed to retool, refocus, and get my life together. I was not doing well in school, having spent so much time on the road to my out-of-town job. And my brand-new marriage needed some tending to, as well. I calmed my fears by telling myself that this was a temporary sabbatical from the pursuit of my dreams.

As part of getting my school career back on track, I had to find an internship. I felt a little silly applying to a television station for a job; now that I had been paid to report, how could I go and work in an unpaid capacity, doing jobs that I thought were clearly below my skill level? Instead I decided to apply at a local radio station. Our broadcasting program had little in the way of hands-on radio training, and I thought it would be good to try my hand at it. Plus the station was only twenty minutes from my house, a far cry from the huge commute of the television station. In the end I thought it would be an easy way to earn my internship credits and possibly learn a bit as well.

I ended up staying for five years.

The station had an oldies format on its FM side, and a sister AM station played adult contemporary music. At first all I had to do was log commercial times and help answer phones, nothing at all to do with actual broadcasting. But it didn't take long to meet and get to know all the nice people who worked there, most of whom were more than willing to show me around the soundboard. Once my bosses learned of my news experience, I was given the chance to give morning news reports on the AM station. I had to get up at the crack of dawn, but I felt once again like I was doing something I was meant to—reporting and announcing news. And it was radio, so my appearance didn't matter! How refreshing that was—I could show up and not feel so self-conscious about how I looked. After the internship was over, I was offered a full-time job, making very little money. They wanted me to do news reports for both the AM and FM stations in the morning and then handle the station's public affairs responsibilities. Another full-time job, and I wasn't even out of college. I felt very lucky, even though I still viewed the situation as temporary. After all, I wanted to be a television reporter—radio didn't make my pulse quicken. And news, to me, was only big in pictures, not just words. Still, I took the job and was excited to be back on the air.

I graduated college and was as heavy as I'd ever been, approaching 250 pounds. Focusing on my classes and the shorter commute to the radio station didn't help my situation as I'd hoped they would. I still overate and didn't exercise, always promising to do better the next day. With my degree in hand, I felt pressured more than ever to hurry up and get my television career restarted—but I couldn't get myself going on any significant weight loss. I stayed at the radio station and right after graduation they added to my duties: They wanted me to cohost the morning show on the FM oldies station.

I was twenty-three years old. It was strange, to me, to be on an oldies station. I had nothing against Elvis Presley or the Beatles, but that was my dad's music. Plus I was a newswoman—I never really saw myself as a laugh-and-cackle morning gal who told jokes and spun tunes. But it was a job, and I was in no shape to look for another one. Plus they gave me the title of news director, and I was still able to do the news for both stations. Again telling myself it was only temporary, that I would do it only until I could lose the weight and get a "real" job, I took it.

The job was a lot of fun. My on-air partner, Larry Smith, was one of the nicest guys you could ever meet, and we had a great rapport. Off air he totally supported my reporting ambitions and always tried to encourage me to lose the weight and get back in the TV game. He was the consummate radioman, and that show meant a great deal to him. I have a lot of guilt about not supporting him in his dreams. You see, on the one hand, being on the radio was great for someone like me: I had a nice voice, and I found it easy to laugh and joke on the air with my buddy Larry. We built an audience, and I had my share of fans, particularly male listeners who would call and talk about how beautiful I sounded and how they would love to see what I looked like. The fact that they couldn't see me allowed me to live in a sort of fantasy world, where I was beautiful and desirable.

But eventually fantasies die and reality sets in. In order for our morning show to grow, we needed to promote it—to hit the streets and meet our listeners in person. I was scared to death. I honestly felt those loyal fans would take one look at me and never listen to our show again. The fantasy would be over, and everyone would know the reality of what I had become physically. I couldn't handle the humiliation, so I refused to help promote the show. I used the excuse that they were paying me peanuts, and really, that was the truth. The extra hours I would have spent making appearances would have gone unpaid. But the people who tuned in every morning and supported our show deserved more, and I certainly owed it to Larry to help him in every way he had helped me. In the end I couldn't face it, and the show suffered, as did our friendship. We lasted several years, and we're still friends today, but I will always regret how I handled that situation (add that to the big pile, I suppose).

I wasn't having much success in the weight-loss department, but I never gave up hope that I would make it back onto TV. I also wasn't getting any younger, and I started to worry that if I didn't do something soon, I was going to lose my window of eligibility. There's no written rule that older women can't be television reporters, just as there is nothing in writing that says overweight women can't be on TV. But I think it's safe to say the deck is definitely stacked against heavier and/or older females.

Then I saw an opportunity to get back into TV—not as an on-air reporter, but with a station I greatly loved and admired.

It was an entry-level position at the Fayetteville bureau of WRAL-TV, the CBS affiliate out of Raleigh/Durham, where Michael had worked as a news photographer for the last several years. I knew I could go in and wow them with my skills. I figured once I lost the weight they would gladly put me on the air. I know this all sounds so unrealistic, but to me, it was quite real and within my grasp. My afternoon job would be in Michael's office, supporting the stories that he and his reporter were working on. I would be doing double duty, because I still worked at the radio station early in the morning. My schedule would be packed, but I figured that was a good thing; no time to eat, right? Right.

Being back in television felt like home. News was my primary focus, and it was where I felt my strengths were. And I worked for an awesome station, with some of the best reporters in the business. I learned so much about news gathering and ethics and journalism, there was no doubt this was my passion. I gave up the radio job so that I could work full-time as an assignment editor at the main station in Raleigh. It was a two-hour commute every day, but I loved it, and I honestly felt it was a means to an end. I still, even after all of that time, felt I would lose the weight and make it on the air. I was already impressing everyone with my work; once I got my appearance in order, I would be well on my way.

The job was wonderful, but it was very stressful. I was in charge of the assignment desk, which is the nucleus of the television newsroom. I helped decide what stories we were going to cover and how we would cover them; I reacted to breaking news with our many resources, including satellite trucks and a helicopter. I had to manage a staff of reporters and photographers and find content for multiple newscasts a day plus our 24/7 news Web site. It was a busy, busy time. I should have lost weight with no problem. But again I used the stress and the commute to my disadvantage, turning to food to calm me down and pass the time riding home. Every day I sent reporters out on stories that I knew I could cover well, that I could tell in a meaningful way. But I just couldn't seem to make it happen. I was beginning to finally face reality: My dream of returning to on-air reporting was starting to slip away.

And then something really strange happened. Our television station also had an FM radio station that played adult contemporary music and had a locally produced morning show. The news was provided by anchors at the television station, which was a hard thing to manage. Those anchors had speaking engagements and other responsibilities, so making it in to do radio in the morning was difficult. Word got around that I had worked in radio for years, and I was asked if I wanted to fill in. I would be paid overtime, which was excellent money, plus I would be able to return to on-air reporting. I was thrilled! I filled in several times and was complimented by many people. The extra money was terrific, and it was exciting to be back on the air.

All of a sudden, though, there was a problem. When I did these newscasts, they were live, from a booth at the television station. I wore headphones, and I plugged in and waited for my cue, much like I had done for years at the oldies station in Fayetteville. But then one day I found myself really, really nervous. This perplexed me. I had done this so many times before, not just at the oldies station, but here for the big station, too.

Why was I scared? But as the commercials wrapped up and the music started to play for my intro, my heart was pounding and my palms were sweating. I went to speak, and I barely had any breath. I sounded truly rattled on the air—it was clear something was wrong. I finished as fast as I could, and the phone immediately rang. It was the morning show crew from their studio across town wanting to know if I was okay. I didn't know what to tell them—I myself couldn't explain what had happened. I just made something up—told them I lost track of time and had to run to the booth and was out of breath. They bought the excuse just fine and said they'd "see" me at my next cut-in, which was in thirty minutes.

I tried to calm myself down, but nothing worked. As the next newsbreak approached, I thought I would pass out from the lack of oxygen; I was that scared. The commercials ended, the music cued . . . and I froze. I couldn't say anything. I turned off my mike and listened to the few seconds of horrible silence in my headphones before the radio crew dumped out and went to commercial. I was stunned. I could not believe what had happened—and worse, I couldn't figure out what to tell them. The phone rang again, and I didn't have to fake a feeble voice when I answered. I lied, saying I'd thrown up right before air-time and couldn't make it back. They sympathized and said they hoped I felt better. I was so relieved there were no more scheduled cut-ins for that morning; there was no way I could face that fear again.

I struggled with that stage fright for the next several months. Sometimes I filled in and was perfectly fine; other times, without any real explanation, I was scared out of my mind. No one ever said anything to me, but I finally couldn't take it anymore. The stress and the fear were too much, and I told my boss that the extra hours were just too hard. I no longer wanted to fill in. Once again my on-air career was over.

It was around this time that I seriously started to realize I would never make it back on the air. I was heavier than ever, now approaching three hundred pounds. I was also getting close to thirty years old, and I should have been getting street-reporting experience for a good ten years by now. And with the unexplained stage fright, I started to consider that this dream just wasn't going to happen. It made me incredibly sad.

I still loved journalism, though, and I excelled at my job on the assignment desk. I was promoted to assignment manager, and I developed real leadership skills that were noticed by my superiors. I started to consider a career in news management, possibly becoming a news director one day. It was a lofty goal, but I felt I had the skills and drive to pull it off. Plus my weight didn't matter.

Or did it?

As I made my way in the corporate world, I was more self-conscious about my size than ever. It undermined my self-confidence, and I believe it kept me from pursuing opportunities. Again, when you have a weight problem, you are screaming to the world that you have issues. There is no hiding the fact that you have a problem. I constantly wondered and worried about what others thought about me, and I was very paranoid. That worry kept me from doing as well as I could have. So much of making it in business and management is political. You have to know the right people and make good impressions. You're constantly thrust into situations where you have to be "on" . . . where you have to exude confidence, even when you don't necessarily feel it. As I slowly moved up the ranks, I found myself invited out to lunch with the head honchos, and I can't tell you how incredibly self-conscious I was. First, I never knew what to order. I felt if I ate modestly, I would draw more attention to myself, like whom was I kidding? A chef salad? Yeah, right! And I always worried about the seating arrangements—just sitting next to people at a table made me feel so big and awkward. And Lord help me if there was a booth I had to squeeze into. Hard to be full of confidence when the table is jabbed into your huge stomach, or God forbid, when others are watching as you try to slide your big ass off the vinyl seat at the end of the meal. It sounds funny, and I suppose I can find some humor in it now, but trust me—back then, it was terrifying.

I was really good at my job, but I was horrible at the social responsibilities that go along with making it in business. I would avoid the company Christmas party every year. What in the world was I to wear? It was a black-tie affair, and most of my female coworkers would arrive in strapless gowns with slits up to there and stilettos. The only size-24 options for me were grandmother-of-the-bride-type selections. One year I found a black and gold long-sleeved sequined jacket and a long black velvet skirt. The jacket was kind of low cut, and I had to buy a special bra to try to create some somewhat attractive cleavage. Truly, I just wanted to crawl under a rock, but I knew I had to go, so I made the best of it. As I got ready for the evening, I tried to convince myself I was young and beautiful and glamorous, but the reality was anything but. The special bra nearly cut off my circulation, and the acts of contortion I had to perform to get into the shimmery off-black Just My Size pantyhose were nothing short of breathtaking. I tried not to be bitter as I considered the fact that the entire outfit cost me almost $500, and I didn't even want to go! I spent the evening smiling and laughing and trying to talk to all the right people. But inside I was mourning the fact that I was dressed way beyond my twenty-eight years—and trying to ignore that I was about to pop out of my 3X top.

The price of being fat was sky-high for me in so many ways. It had robbed me of my dream of being an on-air news reporter. When I settled for wanting to make it in news management, my size kept me from feeling the confidence I needed in order to succeed. As I failed in my career, suffered in my marriage, and started wanting nothing more than to hide from the entire world, I began to realize there was no hiding, no escape. Being morbidly obese affects every single aspect of your life. And to me, there was no way out.

4

The Tale of Three Weddings

The dress didn't fit.

I'm pretty sure that ranks at the top of the nightmare list for every bride-to-be. For months leading up to the big day, we sweat every detail: Should we serve chicken or beef? Will a DJ be enough, or should we splurge and hire a band? Can I get away with seating my future cousins-in-law with crazy Great Aunt Lucille? We make lists, we research bridal magazines, and we consult experts, trying to make sure it's a day everyone will always remember. I was no exception in this regard; after five years with an absolute toad, I'd found my Prince Charming, and I couldn't wait to become Mrs. Joyner. Like all girls, I'd always dreamed of a fairy-tale wedding, and my gown was the centerpiece of that fantasy. Because I got married in the early 1990s, bigger was definitely better, and the dress I picked out was long and flowing in a sea of ruffles and satin and tulle. In my mind I was going to be a vision.

There was one slight problem. Six weeks before the big day, I resigned myself to the awful truth: I couldn't fit into my wedding dress. Not even close. And no amount of alteration was going to solve the problem.

My wedding was toward the beginning of my weight gain— I was bordering on 180 pounds, and I was in an absolute panic.

When I picked out my gown eight months before the event, I felt sure that I could lose the weight necessary to get into the size-12 dress. After all, what better motivation could I find than looking good for my own wedding? I just knew that I could buckle down and do whatever it took to make my dreams come true.

Of course that didn't happen. It was my sophomore year of college, and I was taking a full load of courses. I'd recently landed the on-air reporting job in Florence, which meant I spent three days a week commuting more than three hours. And the wedding I was trying to plan, on my own, was two hours away from where I lived. And we all know how I handled stress.

As the wedding drew near, I took drastic steps. I would vow to fast for several days during the week, only allowing myself to drink liquids and eat Popsicles. When the hunger drove me mad, I would alter the plan, restricting my diet to about 250 calories a day. Of course this strategy was disastrous and only led me to binge eat out of starvation and frustration. Six weeks before the wedding, I could deny it no longer—the dress just didn't fit.

Here's where my saint of a mother came in. She should have been furious. She should have let me have it on both sides for being so irresponsible, but she's not built that way. When I tearfully told her on the phone that the dress wasn't going to work, she soothingly talked me down, assuring me it would be all right. And it was, at least for a little while. The next day she called with the great news: Her best friend's daughter was willing to loan me her wedding dress. It was a size 16, so it should be plenty big, my mom told me. I'd been to her wedding, and I remembered the dress as being quite beautiful. She and I were about the same height, so I knew the length would work just fine. It was awful to think I would not be able to wear the gown I'd chosen for myself, that I would have to rely on the charity of others for one of the biggest days of my life. But I pushed those disappointments away, realizing I really had no other choice. Of course I didn't tell my mom that I had recently started buying work clothes in size 18; my size 16s were getting a little snug. *No problem,* I told myself. *I'll lose just a little weight, just to be sure. No problem.*

I had six weeks before hundreds of my friends and family would gather to watch me exchange vows with the man of my dreams. My parents were spending thousands of dollars on my wedding, and I wasn't sure I would have a dress to wear. Sure, I had a backup plan, but who really knew if it was a realistic one? I had to work every weekend leading up to the wedding; my new reporting job would only allow me a few days off for a honeymoon—there was no extra time. My weekdays were spent in classes, and I simply couldn't make the two-hour trip home to try on the dress. In my moments of panic, I assured myself it would fit, that everything would be all right. Surely this had happened before—surely I wasn't the first bride to do this, right? When my breathing got harder and my head got dizzy, I would have a little something to eat to settle my nerves, promising myself that I would do better the next day.

I lost zero pounds before my wedding.

I finally made it home the Thursday night before the Saturday evening ceremony. You would think the first thing I would do would be to rush right over to try on the dress, making sure that it was going to work. In fact my mom's friend was going to bring the dress right over, but I feigned an excuse, saying I was meeting friends who were coming into town. I just couldn't face it—I was terrified at the thought of the dress not fitting, so I buried it away and refused to deal with it. My mom looked a little worried, but as I walked out the door I assured her it would all be fine.

I needed to try on the dress, but I couldn't make myself. I was scared to death, and I just didn't want to know. *But you're going to have to know sooner or later!* that rational voice inside my head insisted. But once again, rational thinking was not at play.

Friday dawned, and a full day of activities stretched before me: final trip to the florist, lunch with out-of-town guests, quick trip to the mall for some last-minute bridesmaid's gifts. I had a lot to do, many things to keep my mind occupied, but this overwhelming feeling of dread filled every minute. My powers of denial were no longer working, and the bad feeling in the pit of my stomach was growing with intensity. By the time we got to the rehearsal, I was a mess. The mood was jovial as family members greeted one another and everyone congratulated Michael and me. But all I could think about was the next day's wedding and how the bride wore . . . what? Whatever I could find on the rack at Dress Barn? Because in my mind, there was no way that gown was going to fit.

The rehearsal dinner provided a warm and relaxed atmosphere, except in my mind. I didn't touch the prime rib, finally finding whatever it took to refrain from stuffing my face. Too bad that didn't happen three months earlier! The rising panic had made it past the pit of my stomach and was sitting in my throat like hot bile I couldn't swallow away. Michael kissed me and fed me a piece of the chocolate groom's cake to everyone's applause. I wanted to vomit, my fear was so palpable.

I wished Michael a goodnight as he set out to be with his friends, and my girlfriends gathered at the hotel where the reception would be held. We were debating exactly how to spend my last hours as a free woman, when I made up an excuse to go see my mother. I couldn't bring myself to admit to these friends that I had to go figure out what to wear to my wedding the next day; I was too ashamed and embarrassed to admit my failures, even to my closest girlfriends. I don't even remember what I told them, but the next thing I knew, I was on my parents' doorstep at midnight.

"Moooom," I couldn't even get her name out when she opened the door. I sobbed as she hugged me, and like always, she worked her magic. "It's the dress, isn't it?" Of course she knew. She was Mom, and she knew me well. I was crying too hard to answer her, so I just nodded, and she took my hand, leading me to my old bedroom.

The dress hung on the back of the closet door. My mom had steamed it and poofed it, making it all ready for me to wear. Through tears I stripped down and waited for her to bring it to me. In silence I stepped into the dress, and she slowly shimmied the fabric up to my waist. We both held our breath.

It didn't fit.

She couldn't even get the zipper halfway up. As the reality hit us, a strange calm fell over me. So this was it. I had feared this for so many weeks, and at least now I knew: I couldn't fit into my wedding dress. It was almost a relief to let go of the unknown.

While I was imagining what I would say in the hundreds of phone calls I had to make to cancel the wedding, my mom was busy looking at the side panels of the dress. "I think I can let it out," she said quietly, studying the fabric. My breath caught. Had I heard her correctly? Of course I had. This was my mother; she fixed everything! I felt relief wash over my body as she pulled, tucked, examined, and decided what had to be done. I hugged her so tightly and thanked her profusely. She gave me a tired smile, and I couldn't help but note the bit of sadness in her eyes. She sent me off to have a good night's sleep so that I would be beautiful the next day. She would stay up half the night to make it all okay.

I left her house and went straight to the drive-thru.

Some things never change.

The dress did fit the next day, Mom made sure of that. But I was terribly self-conscious about it. You would be hard-pressed to find a photo that does not have me clutching my large bouquet in front of my midsection. I used those flowers as a shield, trying to protect prying eyes from seeing what was happening to me, to my body. When I think back to our wedding, I should be filled with warm memories of dreams finally becoming a reality. Instead all I can recall is heaps of tension, mounds of stress, and tremendous relief that I was at least able to go through with it, that I did not have to cancel my wedding at the last minute because of a wardrobe malfunction.

When the wedding and honeymoon were over and Michael and I began to settle into our lives, the weight gain only increased. The more I tried to stop it, the more I felt as though I were in quicksand. Just living my everyday life was difficult, carrying around all this extra weight I didn't know what to do with. It was bad enough I had to go to school and to work heavier than I'd ever been; I certainly didn't want to let my friends and family back home know that I was spiraling out of control. I started avoiding trips to Durham, too ashamed to see the girlfriends I'd grown up with. Of course I should have confided in them, perhaps they would have even been able to help. I certainly could have used some shoulders to cry on. But my best friends were two of the most beautiful girls you've ever seen, and I foolishly thought they wouldn't be able to understand. How could they identify with my looking worse than I ever had and being unable to do anything about it? Instead of seeing them in person, I kept in touch by phone, never letting on that I was getting fatter by the day.

That was all well and good until a year after my wedding, when my friend SuLin announced her engagement. Because I hadn't been home, I had yet to meet her boyfriend, now fiancé, but I was still so very happy for her and readily accepted her invitation to be one of her bridesmaids. Standing up for SuLin in her wedding as an obese woman was never an option for me; I wouldn't even entertain the notion of walking down an aisle in a gown, well over two hundred pounds. The wedding was several months away, and once again, I stupidly convinced myself that I would be able to look fabulous in a dress by that time. Of course I remembered how my own wedding dress disaster turned out, but I used that as ammunition to try and get myself amped up for this very important weight loss. *I can't let my best friend down! Time to buckle down and do what has to be done.*

I made an excuse when SuLin tried to get me to come home and meet her intended. I feigned work when she asked me to go with her to pick out our bridesmaids gowns. These were fairly simple deceptions to pull off; we lived far apart, and we were both busy with school and work. But when she called asking for my measurements so that she could order my dress (red! strapless!), I could hide no longer. It had already been a couple of months since SuLin had told me she was getting married, several weeks in which I was supposed to have gotten busy with my weight loss. Had it happened? Of course not! What the hell was I going to do now?

I should have come clean, right then and there. I could have confided in SuLin about my continued weight gain and my inability to do anything about it; she was my friend. We'd known each other since fifth grade and had seen each other through some pretty tough times. She would have understood, would have helped me through it. She certainly deserved to know the truth as it pertained to her special day, but I couldn't bring myself to say the words, couldn't admit my failure. *I'll be able to fix it,* I told myself. I came too close to ruining my own wedding, there's no way I'll ruin hers!

I puffed myself up with plans for drastic weight loss, and I gave SuLin *phony* dress measurements. Yes, you read correctly: I completely lied. One of my bridesmaids had been a size 12, and I found her measurements in my wedding planner. I sized them up just a bit to make myself about a size 14. Seriously, at this point I was a size 20 or larger. SuLin's wedding was a mere four months away—a miracle would have to happen in order to get me in that dress. But I somehow convinced myself that telling the truth was way worse than risking letting my best friend down in a huge way; it was easier to try to take it all on my shoulders and make it okay.

Gaining weight and being unable to stop it was one thing; lying about it and in effect sabotaging my best friend's wedding was just inexcusable. If I'd stopped to listen to that inner voice, the one that was screaming at me to stop the nonsense and tell the truth, things would have been a whole lot better for all those involved. But doing so at that point would have meant admitting failure, and I wasn't ready, wasn't able to do that. I had to believe that I could lose this weight, that I could rid myself of this problem. Thinking otherwise, to me, would have meant giving up, and I just couldn't face the failure.

I tried, I really did. I was able to lose a few pounds by watching what I ate and exercising. If I were on a reasonable timetable, maybe I would have had a shot at substantial weight loss. But with each passing day, my panic grew, and the weight wasn't coming off fast enough. *I'll just have to try harder, take more drastic measures,* I told myself. I severely limited my food intake, or tried to fast altogether. But we all know these things don't work, not in the long term. After a few days of starving myself, I would binge eat everything in sight. Net weight loss: zero.

In order to keep up my charade, I had to make up an excuse not to attend SuLin's wedding shower. She wasn't stupid; she had figured out by now that something was really, really wrong. I hadn't yet made arrangements to pick up my bridesmaid's dress, to see if it needed altering. Little did she know that dress could get all the altering in the world; I still wouldn't be able to wear it. I had also promised SuLin she could borrow my wedding veil, and she was waiting to see me in order to try it on and make sure it worked with her dress. I was missing all the festivities leading up to the most important day in my best friend's life. I couldn't believe this was happening, and more important, I couldn't figure a way out.

Finally, about a month before the wedding, I couldn't deny it any longer. I wrote SuLin a letter. I was such a coward, so ashamed, I couldn't even bring myself to tell her on the phone. I did at least tell the truth in writing, letting her know that my weight had been spiraling out of control and I would be unable to stand up for her. As lame as it seemed, I apologized for lying to her, and I truthfully wrote that I didn't know what was happening to me or how to stop it. I told her I loved her, and I sent her the letter, along with the veil.

She called a couple of days later, but of course I was too chicken to pick up the phone. She left me an angry, tearful message, questioning how I could do this to her. I had no excuse, nothing I could say, but I should have tried. She deserved so much better than she got from me. I didn't return her call. I paid for a bridesmaid's dress I never saw, much less wore. And I missed my best friend's wedding. I had made such a mess of things, and I had only myself to blame.

About a year later I heard from SuLin. Incredibly, she missed me and wanted to know how I was. I eagerly called her back and learned her great news: She and her husband were expecting their first child. I cried, happy for her, relieved at her forgiveness, and in sorrow for missing so many important things. She didn't ask me about my weight, sensing (correctly) that I wasn't ready to talk about it. We promised to get together soon. But it never happened. I was by this point morbidly obese and so ashamed of how I looked. I couldn't bear to see SuLin again, and we slowly lost touch. My weight gain, and my inability to deal with it with any sense of rationality, had cost me one of the great friendships of my life. I wasn't sure I'd ever get over it.

If I said the very same scenario almost repeated itself a few years later, surely no one would believe me. There's no way I could have allowed another friend to suffer because of my inability to admit the truth, is there?

Remember who we are dealing with here.

My other best friend, Valerie, was not friends with SuLin, so she missed the entire wedding fiasco. And of course I didn't confide in her what had happened—the fewer people who knew about my horrible weight gain and the destructive path it was taking in my life, the better. As luck would have it, Valerie was in college several hundred miles away from me, and the chances to actually see her were few and far between. We kept in touch by phone, and when it was time for her to walk down the aisle, she asked me to be in her wedding. This was a few years after the SuLin incident and several years into my weight battle. I was close to 250 pounds, and again, the idea of slipping into a bridesmaid's dress was as foreign to me as becoming the queen of England. But of course, I told Valerie I would be in her wedding. I reasoned with myself that I would be more realistic with my weight loss goals this time—I would never try to pretend to Valerie that I could fit into a size-14 dress. Instead I gave her measurements for a size-18 gown, figuring I'd surely be able, this time, to lose some weight. Never mind I was in size-22 work clothes at this point. Never mind that

I already knew Valerie's bridesmaid's dresses were strapless, but mercifully, in navy blue this time around. Could I imagine myself wearing a sleeveless dress at a public event of any sort weighing as much as I did? Heavens, no—and I thought that, along with the humiliation and shame that had accompanied what had happened with SuLin, it would finally give me what I needed to lose the weight.

Shockingly that didn't happen.

Amazingly, though, history didn't completely repeat itself. With two months to go before the wedding, I found the courage to confess my predicament to my friend. In an actual phone call, even. Valerie was upset, angry that I had lied to her. But she was also sympathetic and wanted to help me. She drove to see me the very next day.

Agreeing to see her face-to-face was so hard. I had hidden for so long from the people in my past, even friends who had meant so much to me. But the shame of my actions and my desire to somehow rectify them gave me the strength to face her. She came to my house, and we hugged forever. "You're beautiful," she beamed, and I cried with relief. I had my friend back, and I'd managed to scrape together a bit of integrity.

Being in Valerie's wedding was one of the most difficult things I have ever done. I was never the type to think "big is beautiful," not as it pertained to my own body. I was ashamed, and I felt gross, but I was determined to be there for my friend's big day. I went to see the seamstress, who properly measured me and told me I could possibly fit into a size-24 dress, if we could let it out. I choked back tears as I called the boutique and painfully relayed my dilemma. A couple of days later, I received the bad news: They didn't make the dress in a size 24. The largest was an 18.

Horrified and humiliated, I consulted the seamstress, who found a solution: I could order another size-18 dress, and she could make it work. Yes, I would have to have a dress specially made in order to fit my big fat body. I truly wanted to die, wanted to avoid this public embarrassment at any cost. But I simply couldn't do that to another friend. I had to do whatever it took to make it right, even if it meant losing some face.

The dress was constructed. I was in the wedding. It was really, really hard. I saw a bunch of people I hadn't seen in years, friends who had no idea about my huge weight gain. I smiled and acted as though nothing was wrong. They did the same. My heart was breaking inside, finally having to face the disappointment I had imagined all those years. I felt so very low.

But the smile on Valerie's beautiful face was radiant. She was gorgeous on any day, but on this occasion, she was breathtaking, and I was happy I was there to witness it. I was there for my friend, no matter the cost. And that really did mean something to me.

Like so many other areas of my life, I used my weight gain as an excuse to mishandle the friendships in my life. I lost touch with so many important people, all because I couldn't admit the truth about who I was or was too ashamed to show myself in public. My weight battle left an ocean of regret in its wake, and even as I write this today, I don't know that I will ever truly recover from my own disappointment.

5

Vanity Is a Luxury I Can't Afford

I guess now is as good a time as any to tell you about mooning my in-laws.

Yes, you read that right.

It was way back in 1996. Michael and I had been married for three years, and I was hopelessly entrenched in my weight battle. I don't remember exactly how much I weighed, but I'm thinking it must have been about 240 or so. I say that because on the day in question, I was wearing shorts. I feel pretty confident that once I hit the 250 mark (and beyond), shorts were not something I ever wore in public. Perhaps this incident is the reason why.

Michael and I had just gotten a new puppy, a cute little Jack Russell terrier we named Sasha and who still lives with us today. We were excited to show Michael's parents, so we brought her over to their house. We were all in the family room, sitting on the floor, admiring the new snow-white addition to the family. Michael excused himself for a moment to use the restroom. As soon as he left the room, Sasha stopped jumping and playing on the floor and acted as if she might squat and pee right there on their beautiful rug. Horrified, I jumped up and grabbed her, moving quickly to the back door to take her outside.

And my shorts fell to my ankles.

And. I. Wasn't. Wearing. Underwear.

You see, I was such a hopeless mess about the weight gain and what to do about it that when my underwear no longer fit, I simply stopped buying any. And it didn't help that the shorts I was wearing were from about thirty pounds previous and the elastic was pretty shot. Of course it made no sense, and the shame that I feel now recounting the story is only slightly eclipsed by the sheer horror I felt right in that moment. I froze for about half a second—which felt like an eternity—as I stood at that back door, completely mortified, wondering what in the hell to do. In the end I felt I had no other choice. As deftly as I could, I bent down (aagh!) and picked my shorts back up. Then I walked out the back door, never facing them or seeing their reaction.

And I never spoke of it. Ever.

I never told Michael. And I certainly didn't say anything to my in-laws. I remained outside with Sasha quite a while, and when I came back in, Michael had rejoined his parents. They didn't say a word, and they never indicated they saw anything.

Many of my experiences as an obese person were quite painful and will take years for me to process. But this incident, while embarrassing beyond words, does make me chuckle just a bit. The moral of the story: No matter how much you weigh, if you're planning to go commando, make sure your shorts fit!

They say hindsight is twenty-twenty, and I'm sure all of us can think of several things we'd like to go back and change in our lives. I certainly would love to have not experienced such a huge weight gain, with all its implications. But even within that struggle, I see so many ways in which I didn't help matters, and in some cases, I made them much, much worse.

For example, clothes. When I was a teenager, I was such a clotheshorse. I worked in a department store, and I used my discount to buy beautiful jackets and sweaters and suits. I always dressed older than my age, and I was usually overdressed, even at school. But I loved it. I enjoyed looking professional, even as a young adult. And I loved picking out clothes and trying new combinations.

I suppose you could say I was overcompensating. I was always overweight, and I never felt pretty or admired. Clothes were my way of looking as nice as I possibly could, and I took great pride in what I wore. I may have been chubby, but I was neat and stylish!

When the added weight gain started, I was barely in my twenties. At first I just bought bigger sizes. It hurt to have to do so, but remember: I always had a plan, always had a strategy as to how I was going to fix it. When I had to start buying clothes in sizes 14 and 16, I figured it was only temporary. But of course it didn't get better, and soon size 16 didn't fit. And then size 18 didn't fit. And I was completely lost and devastated. When this happened to me, in the early 1990s, there wasn't the proliferation of plus-size clothing there is now. Obese women had to shop at stores like Catherine's, a place I remember going to with my grandmother when I was a little girl—a place that, back then, definitely catered to the over-sixty crowd. There was no Lane Bryant. No Ashley Stewart. I was relegated to the misses section at department stores like Ivey's and Belk, where I had limited choices. I may have dressed older than my age, but the clothing options left to me were for the geriatric set. So not only was I gaining weight and feeling terrible about my inability to do anything about it, I was also unable to make myself feel better with stylish clothes, something that had always helped me when I struggled with weight issues growing up.

Shopping for a special occasion was a nightmare, and I avoided it as much as possible by simply not attending special occasions. I made excuses when it came to company holiday parties or special birthday events. But sometimes I just couldn't avoid it. My brother-in-law's mother died after a long battle with cancer, and it was important to me to be there for the funeral. The problem: I had nothing to wear. You would think a black outfit would have been easy to come up with, but everywhere I looked, the clothes were fitted jackets and skirts for size-4 women. Finally, after a long day of store hopping, I found what can only be described as a big black tent that masqueraded as a dress. Sure it had little fancy gold buttons and a collar, but it was a size-24 black bedsheet as far as I was concerned. Still, I had to have something, and it fit, so I bought it. I wore it to work the next day before the funeral, and one of my coworkers walked in and said, "Hey! It's Mama Cass!" You know, from the Mamas and the Papas? Yeah, not very complimentary, unless you have a great singing voice. I don't. I choked back tears and thought about how that's what I got when I tried to make an effort.

So, I just gave up.

I was tired from looking, and I wanted to do anything to avoid the pain I felt when I shopped, so I didn't shop. I bought three to four outfits that I could fit into, and that was all I wore. No, I didn't think that was okay, but again, the push-pull was always at play. I would convince myself that my state was temporary and I would soon be in more normal clothes sizes.

Over the years, as obesity numbers in this country sky-rocketed, the clothing choices got better. You had labels that catered to plus-size women without giving up (too much) fashion. Even well-known brands like Liz Claiborne and Tommy Hilfiger designed clothing for larger ladies. But I, sadly, never caught on. I should have, no matter my size, taken more pride in my appearance. But honestly I couldn't stand to look in the mirror. I absolutely detested shopping for clothes because it made me confront, head-on, how much weight I had gained and how much I had lost because of my weight. Clothes used to be such a source of pleasure for me, and now the weight and my inability to control it had robbed me of that enjoyment.

Now that's not to say I never bought anything. I was a professional career woman, and I had to have clothes for work. But I kept it as safe and as bland as possible. First of all, I had every variation of the black top available. Black sweater. Black blouse. Black button-down shirt with long sleeves. Black turtle-neck. I wore so much black that my brother once referred to me as Johnny Cash (ouch). And Michael's grandmother once took me by surprise when several family members were talking about their favorite color. She said my favorite color must be black because I wore it all the time (ouch again). No, black wasn't my favorite color, but it's what I thought I needed to wear to hide as much as I possibly could. I had a few pairs of slacks that I rotated around to go with my various black tops, but truly I only had four to five working outfits at any given time. I just couldn't bring myself to buy more. I stupidly thought that doing so would be admitting defeat, and if I couldn't buy all the beautiful clothing I wanted in the sizes I longed for, then I wasn't going to buy pretty clothes at all. I really made it so much worse than it needed to be. But what can I say? I was mired in sickness. After years of mightily battling my weight, and failing miserably, I think I convinced myself that I didn't deserve to look good, that it was pointless to spend time and money on my appearance. My self-worth took such a beating; instead of making the most out of a bad situation, I chose to wallow in my misery. Not only did I feel like crap, I looked like shit most of the time.

When I could no longer fit into 3X clothing, I was forced to go to more of the specialty shops. This was when I was approaching three hundred pounds, and department stores tend to stop at size 24W, or 3X. Thank goodness this didn't happen in the early to mid-1990s, because I don't know what I would have done then, the choices were so limited. But as it was, I could go to Lane Bryant and find bigger sizes. The cost was enormous, but I had no other choice. I do chuckle to myself when I remember one time being in the dressing room, trying on a couple different versions of the black top in size 26/28 (yikes!), when all of a sudden a woman from another dressing room cried out, "It fits!" I think all the women there could relate to the relief in her voice, and we all broke out in spontaneous applause. It was one of the few times that I can remember somewhat bonding with another overweight woman, although it was through the relative anonymity of a closed-door dressing area.

There are two clothing items I abstained from completely as a morbidly obese person: jeans and bathing suits. The latter has to be pretty obvious, I think. I know there are plenty of plus-size women who have no problem wearing bathing suits, refusing to allow extra pounds to keep them from enjoying themselves. I

am so not one of those women. Yes, I have been kn
the beach FULLY CLOTHED. We're talking long
pants—the works—because I couldn't bear the thought of baring it all in public. I think I would have rather died first. I felt
much the same way about jeans. I thought once you reached a
certain size, jeans were no longer an option. And I made that
decision even before "skinny jeans" became so popular. I suppose taking that stance came of out of necessity in the beginning.
Again, there weren't many options when I first started to really
gain weight, and other than buying a pair of husky men's jeans at
Kmart, an obese woman was pretty much out of luck. Of course
that changed over the years, and now you can buy virtually any
size jeans you want; but I still can't make myself do it, even now
that I'm not morbidly obese. I don't know, something seems too
binding about them to me. There have been many, many nights
over the years when I wondered if I would ever put on a pair of
sexy jeans for my husband again, if I would one day don a bathing suit and play at the beach with my kids. When I was deluding
myself, I thought, *No problem, I can easily do that in the next six
months or so.* At my lowest I felt as though jeans and bathing suits
had passed me by forever. Sometimes, I still feel that way.

Ugghh . . . my back aches. Wanna know why? Because I've had
to keep my legs and thighs exactly together all day. Wanna know
why? I have a hole in my pants in the inner thigh area. Now I
guess you want to know why I wore these pants when I knew they
had a hole in them. BECAUSE I CAN'T FIND ANY PANTS

TO FIT ME! I've been shopping at least five times in the last ten days, and I've come up empty. Yes, I have black pants . . . yes, I have gray pants. (Gray! Doesn't that by itself sound terribly depressing?!) But I can't find cream pants or khaki pants . . . and I can't wear the same black pants over and over. In fact I already feel as though I'm doing that, and I am terribly self-conscious about it. So that's why I knowingly wore a pair of pants with a hole in them. And I am now paying the price in backaches.

❧

I wish I could say that kind of thing was rare, but sadly, it wasn't. I was so determined not to confront my appearance issues that I let things like that slide all the time. I can remember blouses with permanent stains on them that I convinced myself weren't that bad and wore them anyway. They *were* that bad. I can also remember taking a shirt out of a dry cleaner's bag and discovering that one of the buttons had been broken in half. I was running late and didn't have anything else clean, so I wore the blouse to work anyway. When you only have three or four blouses to choose from, it really puts you in a bind if something goes wrong. So I told everyone I didn't notice it until I got all the way to work. I tried to laugh it off, but I knew how pathetic I was being.

Being obese makes clothing emergencies all the more difficult. When we went out of town to visit family, I couldn't simply borrow a jacket if I forgot to bring one. No one had anything that fit me, not even the men. When I volunteered in the church kitchen, I couldn't wear one of the standard aprons emblazoned with the church logo because they were too small.

But perhaps the most embarrassing problems occurred when I was faced with unplanned clothing situations at work.

Winters in North Carolina tend to be pretty mild; if we get a good dusting of snow once a year, we're doing pretty well. But in 2002 we had one big snowfall after another, and this meant extra-long hours of work because I was employed by a television news station more than an hour away from my home. Once I was caught off guard; I was still at work when the ice started to build up on the roads, and the forecasters were predicting widespread power outages and road delays. I would have to spend the night, perhaps several nights, in a local hotel so that I could make it into work. Normally this would only be mildly inconvenient, but for someone with a big weight problem, it seemed catastrophic. What was I going to wear? I hadn't packed any clothes, and it looked as though I'd be stuck for several days. Finding clothes to fit me was difficult under the best of circumstances, when I had several stores to choose from; now, I had to go to Kmart, the only store that was open and just down the street, hoping and praying to find something I could wear.

I went first to the women's section, picking out a few simple tops and bottoms in the largest sizes they had—24. I took the clothes to the dressing room and confirmed what I already knew in my heart: The clothes didn't fit. They were too small. Fighting tears, I hung them back on the rack and made my way to the men's section. They had some husky-size sweatshirts and sweatpants in men's 3X. I swallowed hard and took the men's clothes back to the women's dressing room, hoping no one would notice. The clothes fit, but not entirely well. Still though, I had a problem. These were sweat clothes, and the only shoes

I had with me were dress flats. I had to go over to the shoe section and pick out sneakers. I knew I would look ridiculous in these clothes, and I felt so much worse. But what choice did I have? I was stuck, with nowhere else to turn. I got through the next three days the best I could. And I was never caught again in wintertime without an extra set of clothes packed in my car.

ॐ

I have reached a new wardrobe low. Eli's baptism is almost here, and I have nothing to wear. And I don't mean I have nothing that I like; I mean I have absolutely nothing dressy that will fit my body. Going shopping for clothes is right at the top of the list of things I hate to do, along with going to the dentist and having my taxes audited. But this is one special occasion I cannot—I will not—miss.

Nothing would make me happier than to buy a beautiful sundress in a pretty pastel color. It's April, and we're holding the party after the baptism in our backyard. Everywhere you look the colors of spring are bursting, and I'd love to match, or at least come close to matching, the joy of the occasion with my outfit. But pastel and three hundred pounds don't really go that well together, and at the rate I'm going, color is not going to be a privilege afforded to me. I've been to all the major department stores and have come up empty—nothing fits. Fighting back tears, I make my way down to the mall to one of the specialty shops. I should be used to this by now: wanting something to wear for a special occasion and being utterly disappointed by my choices—or lack thereof. But this really hurts. This is my baby boy's baptism. After some initial health problems at birth, he's now thriving at nine months old and cute as all get out. I want to celebrate with my family and friends; I want how I look to reflect how I feel about Eli. But how I look only reflects the inner turmoil that rocks me on a daily basis, and a drab outfit bought in an act of desperation certainly will not help matters.

In the end I settle for a black linen jacket and a hot pink shell to wear underneath. I pair them with the same long black skirt I've worn on many occasions, a skirt that honestly looks like a bedsheet. Dressed in black, in the springtime, at an outdoor party for my baby boy's baptism. Lovely. As unexcited as I am about the outfit, I'm even more depressed at how much the clothes cost me. *At least Michael will have something to bury me in,* I tell myself.

❧

I certainly could have handled it all a whole lot differently, perhaps have even made myself feel better, if I'd simply done all I could to help my appearance. Even if I was heavier than I'd ever been, even if I had to shop high and low for hours on end, I should have made more of an effort. But truly, the reality of how I looked put me into a state of shock. As the weight piled on, there were things happening to me that I never thought possible.

❧

You know how some people have double chins? Well I definitely had those, and I think one extra. But what was really weird is at one point I had three *stomachs*. It was right after my second C-section. I remember my sister-in-law saying her C-section permanently damaged her abdomen, that no matter what she did as far as exercise and diet, she couldn't get her stomach flat again. I scoffed at that notion, especially after my first C-section, in which my stomach went back to its normal (lumpy) state. Nothing looked different to me (unfortunately). But after my second surgery, it did change. I had the same roll of fat above the belly button, you know, right above where you fasten your pants (or for me, tie the drawstring). And then I had the same enormous roll of fat below the navel. But in between the two, I developed a third layer of blubber that added incredible insult to injury. Sucking it in? Not even close to an option, although really, it wasn't much of an option before. Still, I looked like an absolute freak, and it wasn't just my stomach making me feel that way.

About a year after I started gaining weight and was unable to stop it, I started to lose my hair. As I tell this now, it's easier, because it started so long ago and I have since accepted it. But at the time, I was beyond bitter. Was my fate really meant to be this way? Not only was I on my way to morbid obesity, but I was now going to draw even more attention to myself by becoming bald? I panicked. I went to see a specialist. And then another and then another. No one could tell me why it was happening, and there were no suggestions as to what to do about it. Sure, I tried Rogaine. I tried hair supplements and special shampoos. Nothing worked. The pounds piled on, and the strands of hair littered my clothing, my sink drains. I started to get comments from well-meaning coworkers. "Do I see your scalp?" one lady asked me, looking closely at my head. I was mortified, and depressed beyond belief. I was heavier than I had ever been. I wore the same three to four black-blouse outfits every day. And now my hair was thinning. After a while I just grew kind of numb to it all. On better days I would convince myself that once I started to lose the weight, my hair would come back, even though the doctors I saw couldn't tell me if my weight gain had anything to do with it. On my really bad days, I told myself that I already looked like crap and the hair loss just completed the shitty picture. I accepted it as though I deserved it.

I felt like a shell of the young woman I once was. Granted, I was never a beauty queen, but I took pride in looking the best that I could, wearing cute clothes and styling my long auburn brown hair in a pretty decent way. I wasn't bad looking, I told myself. But now I was beyond bad. I bordered on grotesque. And it all seemed to happen so quickly that it took my breath away. The quicker the changes came, the more powerless I felt to do anything about them. When I tried to get motivated to lose weight, I would think, *What's the point? I've got stretch marks covering my body. My hair is gone, and my skin has never looked worse. How can I possibly improve all of this?* And when I tried to find solutions to my hair, perhaps a wig or a weave, I would get discouraged and wonder why I was going to such trouble and expense when I was helplessly—hopelessly—fat. It was a vicious cycle, and I was forever trapped.

The John Hughes film *The Breakfast Club* is one of my favorite movies of all time. In it Judd Nelson's character asks the teenage girl played by Molly Ringwald her name. When she tells him it's Claire, he tells her that's a fat girl's name. "I'm not fat," she protests. But Nelson's character says one day she could be: "You see, I'm not sure if you know this, but there are two kinds of fat people. There's fat people that were born to be fat, and there are fat people who were once thin but became fat. So when you look at them you can sort of see that thin person inside."

Whenever I've watched that movie over the years, especially once the weight started to pile on, I've felt as though Nelson's character was speaking to me. Growing up I was never considered thin. But compared to the morbidly obese, I was certainly on the average side. But that changed, and I felt trapped in a grossly bloated body—an overstuffed version of what I once was—unable to get out, unable to do anything about my health. Unable to live my life.

Even though I kind of gave up on my appearance at times, I constantly worried about what other people thought. The stereotypes of fat people were forefront in my mind, including the notion that all fat people are lazy (no, we're not) and fat people smell. For the longest time I dismissed that as silly. I was heavy, to be sure, but I didn't have any hygiene problems. On *Oprah* I once saw a woman who weighed five hundred pounds admit that she had trouble washing herself. *I'll never be that fat,* I vowed to myself.

You know where this is going.

At my worst I was 336 pounds.

And I had trouble keeping clean.

If you think about it, it makes sense. Your arms are only so long; if your middle keeps growing, sooner or later you're going to have problems reaching all areas. And I did. Admitting this makes me sad beyond words, but it's important to me to be honest, to let others who are suffering know they are not alone. This does happen, and it is devastating, especially to women. How much more basic can you get than your ability, or inability, to wash your body parts? You take a person whose self-esteem already takes a daily beating and then add this to the mix, and you've got a real mess on your hands. Unfortunate pun not intended.

What did I do? Thank the Lord for handheld showers. I tried to sound casual when I mentioned to Michael that I preferred our kids' shower to the one in our bedroom. Really I don't know how he didn't see right through me; we both knew their shower had terribly low water pressure. But it had a handheld shower, and the one in our bathroom did not. I was too ashamed to simply ask Michael to install one in our shower; as it was, I hoped he would never discover the real reason I was using our kids' bathroom. If he ever did figure it out, he never let on, and I love him for it.

It's for these humiliating reasons that I have a hard time believing there are people out there who are happy being overweight. I mean let's forget for a moment about the physical tolls obesity inflicts on your health—the increased risk for diabetes, high blood pressure, joint pain, sleep apnea, heart disease, cancer, and early death rates. What about the daily embarrassments and humiliations you suffer when you are so heavy? You can't fit into a restaurant booth. You break toilet seats. You have to go to extraordinary measures to bathe. Could anyone possibly be happy with that? Some say they are, but I'm sorry, I don't believe it. Maybe saying so is a defense mechanism of some sort, and I can totally sympathize with the need for that.

But the truth is, being morbidly obese is a disgusting, humiliating, torturous existence that threatens your very life. There's nothing to be happy about.

Now does that mean that all morbidly obese people are as miserable as I was? Absolutely not. I think many, many people handle it much better than I did, and I applaud them for it. We only get one life, and we all have challenges to face. I believe it is how we behave in the face of adversity that really defines who we are. And it's that belief, I think, that caused me even more unhappiness. Why couldn't I get it together? What did it say about me that I couldn't care enough about myself to do better, to make the most of a bad situation? I allowed the weight gain and subsequent physical problems to prevent me from maintaining friendships, from seeking career opportunities, from bettering my marriage and my family life. I collapsed under the weight of obesity. I totally lost who I was and all the things I cared about.

It certainly didn't help matters when I developed what I laughingly called "the flesh-eating virus." During my second pregnancy, with my gestational diabetes raging out of control and my body expanding rapidly to accommodate what would become a twelve-pound newborn, I noticed a nasty rash forming under the folds of my skin, right under my belly. It was itchy and bumpy and awful . . . and it smelled rancid. It looked like something out of a horror movie, and nothing I did made it go away or helped the odor dissipate. Finally I showed it to my doctor at a prenatal appointment, and she gently gave me the news: It was a yeast infection. Now I've heard of women developing yeast infections, but never under their stomachs. No, my doctor informed me, this happened because of all the heat and friction in that area of my body.

Shoot. Me. Now.

I had to get a specially prescribed powder, which I applied three times a day. After a shower I had to lie flat on my bed and use a hair dryer to make sure the area was dry at all times. I was beyond mortified, especially when the problem kept coming back after I'd given birth. I was so big and my stomach so large that I frequently developed these types of infections. The fact that my diabetes didn't go away after my pregnancy didn't help; people with diabetes are more prone to yeast infections. Yet another embarrassing problem I inflicted upon myself because I couldn't get my eating under control. I felt like a million bucks.

With every humiliation, every embarrassment, I hoped I would get fed up enough to change my life. Sometimes I did manage to change my habits for a bit, getting my eating under control and bringing my bingeing to a halt. But those successes were rare. Instead I used the bad stuff to further convince myself that I wasn't worthy of looking good, of feeling good about myself. I was stuck in a terrible, vicious cycle. And no matter how hard I tried, I couldn't find a way out.

6

Work It Girl, Phase 10,280

I can remember the exact day I uttered the dumbest string of words ever to leave my lips. It was July 1992, and I had just finished my freshman year of college. I was working part-time in the handbags section of a department store, and my coworkers and I were using the lull in the summer shopping season to discuss the important matters of hair, clothes, and makeup. The talk inevitably turned to weight, and the others started lamenting about how bad they looked in their swimsuits that year. My issues were a bit bigger than beachwear: I had recently gained back a little of the weight I'd lost my senior year of high school—a weight increase I chalked up to being in love with a great guy (finally) and not paying enough attention to what went into my mouth. I admitted to these girlfriends that I was back at my old standby weight of 165—a number on the scale I'd spent most of my teen years trying to permanently ditch. "But at least I know one thing," I proclaimed with certainty. "I eat and eat and eat, and I never go past 165."

If I could reach back in time and yank that stupid girl by the hair, shaking her into reality, I would most assuredly do so.

Within a year of that asinine comment, I would be approaching two hundred pounds.

And, well, we know where I went from there.

I spent most of my adult life daydreaming of being 165 pounds again. Over the years I hatched plan after scheme after program to get me there. I read all the latest diet books. I watched all the current health documentaries. I signed up for nutritional classes, for support groups. I joined walking clubs and fitness centers. I bought fresh new notebooks and filled the pages with detailed eating plans and elaborate exercise charts. I excitedly showed Michael my "Work It Girl, Phase 1 & 2" outline, sure that this time it would work. Over the years, it became a (good-natured) joke between me and my husband: "Work It Girl, Phase 10,280! This is the one!"

I know it's hard for outsiders to believe, but I honestly thought, each and every time, that my latest plan would work. Every diet book, every weight guru drills into us the same theme: "If you are determined, and if you work hard, you will succeed." I approached weight loss as if I were studying for a big exam: I read everything I could get my hands on, I studied caloric charts and memorized fat gram contents, I outlined detailed food intake plans and exercise routines. I put in hours and hours of time, but ultimately I got very little success in return.

I can remember being about eleven years old and desperately wanting to shed my chubby tummy. My brothers teased me endlessly, and the kids at school knew right where to go if they wanted to hurt me: "Fat pig!" was a common retort from my adversaries on the playground. During the summer months I became convinced that all my schoolyard problems would be resolved if I lost a little weight before September.

So there I was, barely a fifth grader, tuning in to the *Richard Simmons Show* every morning. I wrote down eating tips, I listened to the motivational stories, and I sweated to the oldies with the end workout routine. I tried to ride my bike a little more around the neighborhood, and I walked to my friends' houses instead of having Mom drive me. I even tried to cut back on all the chips and soda around the house. Looking back it was a pretty healthy effort at weight loss, save for the fact that I was still in grammar school! I doubt if I lost any real weight, however; all it really did was mark the beginning of a lifelong struggle of desperately trying to combat nature.

※

I've already mentioned the weight loss I did achieve when I was a senior in high school. Truth be told, it was my only successful effort at shedding pounds without the aid of diet drugs or surgery. How did I do it? Where did I find the willpower? If I knew the answer to that, I would have employed it many times over again! All I know is that it was really, really hard. I can remember going to bed early, in tears, because I was so hungry and wanted to eat so badly. I recall forcing myself to drink diet soft drinks and hating every minute of it. But at the end of the effort was the reward: I'll never forget putting on a short black skirt and having men stop and stare at me as I walked down the mall. Yeah—that feeling stands out the most!

After I was married and the weight started to pile on, I tried to find that elusive willpower again. I would go for about two weeks, managing to avoid fast food and sticking to Diet Sprite and baked potato chips. But I always, always fell off the wagon. I'd buy a candy bar and eat it fast before I really had a chance to think about it, or I would give in to temptation and stop at McDonald's. I'd slip up, and I'd allow it to devastate me. I was never able to pick myself up, dust myself off, and keep going. I would instead wallow in self-pity, eating all I wanted, vowing to get it out of my system and then right the wrong. I thought maybe that was the way to go—thinking back to that New Year's Eve when I ate everything and then went on to lose a bunch of weight on my own. I tried to recreate that elusive magic, time and again.

It never happened.

I became convinced I was not in charge. Willpower was a force that was going to be bestowed upon me from Heaven above, and I had to just sit and wait for it to hit. I prayed. I read. I studied. I waited. I felt weak, and I needed help. I thought if I wanted it bad enough, help would just magically appear. I was not the one in control of my destiny.

In the winter of 1997, I reached critical mass. It had been years since I'd had significant weight loss. I was approaching 280 pounds, and I grew panicked. My dreams of being a television reporter were slipping by with each passing day; I wasn't getting any younger, and I thought I had a very narrow window in which to get my career started. Not to mention the toll my now-morbid obesity was taking on my marriage. Michael and I had only been married four years, and he was baffled by what was happening to me. He never once said anything negative to me about my weight—he was more concerned about what it was doing to me, to my self-esteem and quality of life. He wanted to help, but felt powerless and frustrated. I beat myself up daily, wondering why in the world I couldn't get it together.

I went to my ob-gyn for my annual checkup and dissolved into tears as I opened up about my turmoil. She listened patiently as I explained the many ways in which I'd tried to shed the pounds. She ordered a full blood work-up to see if she could find a problem, but in the meantime she had a question for me: Had I ever considered diet drugs?

Up until that point, my thoughts on diet drugs were almost all negative. We've all heard about women getting amped up on Dexatrim or other appetite suppressants bought at the drugstore. We've all seen the episodes of *The Facts of Life* or *Beverly Hills, 90210* in which one of the main characters abuses diet pills and finds herself in trouble. My mom was even part of that elite club. Back when she had me, she said doctors were really tough on women about getting baby weight off quickly after giving birth. They frequently prescribed "black beauties" to help new moms burn off the fat. The pills were *speed!* My mom said they worked great: She lost all her excess weight in no time—and her mind, too—as she stayed up all night cleaning the house, organizing closets, and doing everything else except sleeping. Diet drugs, to me, sounded dangerous and reckless, something I felt I should avoid.

My doctor explained that there was a new combination of drugs called fen-phen, a weight-loss regimen that was seeing a lot of success. These drugs were only prescribed to extremely heavy patients, so the potential of abuse by people who shouldn't be taking them was all but eliminated. Whatever side effects caused by these drugs—and they really weren't sure what those were long-term—were tempered with the great benefit of shedding weight off of morbidly obese patients whose very lives were threatened by their excess pounds. The risk seemed to be justified.

Could this be the answer? Could I solve my problems simply by taking medicine? It seemed doubtful to me, but nothing else was working at that point. My doctor was recommending it, so why not give it a chance? How bad could it be? I agreed to try it, without much hope or expectation.

It was like freedom in a bottle.

The drugs made me not care—about much of anything, really—but specifically, I didn't care about eating. It wasn't that I was *not* hungry per se, I was just indifferent toward food. And that was incredibly liberating. I could go about my day and not obsess over whether I would binge eat fast food; I truly didn't want to. As the weight started to come off, my confidence began to build. For the first time in a long time, I had real hope. The scales were finally going in the right direction, and I felt I had that elusive control I'd fought so hard to find.

People started to notice my weight loss, and that fueled me even further. I began to exercise, and I loved it. I walked for miles around the track at the local high school, listening to Sugar Ray, Smash Mouth, and Third Eye Blind on my Walkman, feeling young, alive, and vital. I daydreamed about finally getting back into reporting, realizing my dream of continuing my on-air career. I was able to take an interest in clothes and start to look forward to buying pretty things again. Life was beginning to feel good once more.

If the drugs had negative side effects, I was unaware. The most discomfort I ever felt was dry mouth, which actually worked in my favor, causing me to drink lots of water and avoid soft drinks. I never felt dizzy or disoriented, never had that heart-racing feeling you sometimes hear about. I became convinced that these drugs were meant for me, that they were the key to reclaiming my life.

I still loved to eat and found that it was okay to do so. I just manipulated the times that I ate around the times I took my medication. For example, if I was craving a particular food, I would plan to have it for breakfast. Sure, spaghetti with meat sauce sounds a little gross first thing in the morning, but it worked for me. I stuffed myself until I was satisfied, then a couple of hours later, I took my pills and was fine for the rest of the day. I didn't obsess over the foods I couldn't have, I just planned them for when I could eat them. I never felt deprived, and most important, the results made me feel fabulous. I couldn't believe I hadn't thought of this solution sooner.

After about eight months, I'd lost fifty-five pounds. I was down to about 230, lower than I'd been in years. My dream of being a television reporter was starting to feel attainable again; I really felt as though I could do anything I wanted to. I hadn't been this excited about the future in a long, long time.

And then the rug was yanked out from under me.

My mom called me at work. It's kind of ironic that I am a self-proclaimed news junkie and like to think I know everything before others, and yet my mother—a decidedly non–news junkie—called *me* with *the news*.

"Jennifer! Did you see the news on Channel 5? They said those diet drugs cause heart damage. They're pulling them off the market!"

I wasn't too worried at first. My mom tended to be kind of alarmist about this kind of thing—not to mention not very accurate. Surely she was wrong; surely the report referred to another kind of diet drug. After all, my doctor had suggested these pills. They weren't dangerous! There had to be a mistake.

There was no mistake. The makers of fen-phen were pulling the drugs off the market after several reports of heart valve damage. Some people had even died.

My immediate reaction was to go into self-protection mode. *Look at how much weight you have lost,* I told myself. *You don't need drugs anymore! You've started to exercise, you've cut down on bad foods, you can do this! The rest of the weight will come off easily!*

It never once occurred to me to be worried about my health. I was twenty-five and felt invincible. My weight—at least in my warped way of thinking—had nothing to do with health and everything to do with vanity. Never mind that I had just spent eight months taking a combination of drugs that some claimed did permanent damage to their hearts. I felt fine! No need to worry about that.

No, my immediate concern was to ensure my future weight loss, to make sure I could continue to drop pounds. And for a little while, I did. I kept up the exercise, and I tried to stay with the same eating habits. Slowly the overwhelming hunger started to creep back in, no matter how hard I pushed it away. I managed to beat it back and maintain what I had lost for about a year. But eventually I succumbed to my never-ending cravings for all things bad. The negativity in my mind really started to do a number on me: *You can't do this by yourself. You tried for years, and look where it got you. The only time you really lost weight was when you had the drugs, when you had help. Don't even try, you will fail.*

The weight came back, and then some. Sure I tried to beat it. Every day I once again started something new, some different way to take control, to do it myself. For example, I once signed up for Weight Watchers. I liked the thought of using everyday, normal food, just in moderation. I had such a limited palate, I thought this would be the eating plan that would work for me. I showed up for the first meeting at the Baptist church in my small town. There wasn't anyone in the room younger than fifty. Embarrassed, I weighed in, in front of everyone, and then sat for the group discussion. All the talk focused around cooking for families and eating sensibly at work. No one talked about obsessing every minute of every day about what they ate. Not one person offered up that they stuffed themselves until they were sick, hiding food in their homes and their cars. I had absolutely nothing in common with the group, and worse, I felt like some sort of freak. I didn't go back.

Another example: When I worked at the radio station, employees were offered free gym memberships through one of its sponsors. I happily signed up, thinking this would be it, this would be what motivated me, what made me turn the corner. As part of the sign-up, I got a free session with a trainer. Great! An expert who could tell me exactly what I needed to do! I was a let's-make-a-plan kind of girl, and this was going to be just the plan I needed.

The trainer was a nineteen-year-old stud named Ricky. He had a hard body and a killer smile, and I was beyond mortified. To make matters worse he acted as though he drew the short straw by having to work with the big fat radio girl. He weighed me (kill me now) and took my body fat measurements (okay, just shoot me). And then he started going over strength-training exercises. Strength training? Did I look like I needed strength training? I feigned a headache and got the hell out of there, making a beeline for the hot dog joint across the street. Again, hot tears spilling down into my food didn't stop me from eating.

I did go back to that gym, sans trainer. But it clearly was not the place for me. All young, beautiful hard bodies were there, trolling for dates just as much as looking to exercise. I was so self-conscious, I couldn't do much of anything.

Now could I have made these two situations better? Of course. I could have kept looking for a Weight Watchers group that worked for me, even if it meant driving to another town. I could have joined another gym, perhaps one that catered to women. Money was certainly an issue (when is it not?), but with the cash I was spending on food, I'm sure I could have scraped up the funds needed. But with every experience like the old lady Weight Watchers or the hard body gym, I just felt more and more defeated. Helpless. Hopeless. Out of time and out of luck.

It was during the really desperate times that I would go back to one idea that refused to go away: gastric bypass surgery. Reading about Carnie Wilson's experience with the procedure and seeing her successful results made a great impression on me, but I was still skeptical. Sure, I felt pretty desperate, but having surgery seemed so drastic to me. When I first started to think it over, I'd never been hospitalized before, never had any sort of surgery. I couldn't imagine willingly going in and allowing doctors to cut away. But the results were undeniable: Al Roker looked fantastic, Carnie Wilson was a knockout, and probably the story that had the most impact on me was Blues Traveler front man John Popper. I caught a VH1 special that detailed his experience and could hardly believe it when he said he'd lost two hundred pounds in a year. Holy crap! After a heart scare, his friends talked him into exploring gastric bypass. He said he thought there was no way he would lose the weight, no way he'd be able to give up McDonald's french fries or Burger King hamburgers. Boy could I relate to that! After having the surgery, though, he couldn't imagine he ever ate at those places. He'd always seen himself as a frog, and now he was slowly becoming a prince.

After watching that special, I was blown away. Was I missing something right in front of my face? I had tried so hard for so long, and I was just watching the years slip away without any solution. Was it finally time to make a permanent change?

In 2002 I thought I was ready. I started off the New Year like I did every January, full of promises and plans to lose the weight and keep it off. I did well for a bit, but then something small and inconsequential sent me straight to the drive-thru. As I polished off two chili cheese dogs and a jumbo bag of fries, I thought about how all my efforts had led to only three days of healthy eating and exercise—how someone saying the wrong thing to me made me throw away all my hard work. I knew I had a problem; I was well aware that I was simply looking for any excuse to overeat, to self-sabotage. Fed up, I vowed then and there that if I didn't do something in the next six months, if I didn't manage to stick to a plan and make significant headway with this problem, then I was making an appointment with a gastric bypass surgeon. I was finally disgusted with myself enough to self-issue an ultimatum—and I meant it.

And then, wouldn't you know it, word started coming out against gastric bypass. Suddenly it wasn't the cure-all everyone had hoped for; for all the Carnie Wilsons and Al Rokers out there, there were plenty of people who suffered serious complications from the procedure. *People* magazine did a piece on it in 2003, profiling several gastric bypass surgeries gone wrong, including a woman who had to have her arm amputated! I used that negative information to climb back onto my high horse about gastric bypass. *That's what happens when people take the easy way out,* I told myself. It seemed like such a good idea: Go to the doctor and have him make it so you can't overeat. Finished, end of story. But of course nothing is as easy as that, and I felt this was proof. I quickly got off of the idea, deciding that I needed to lose the weight "on my own" in order for it to really count.

I knew I was in trouble. I felt sick—and not just from the physical toll of carrying around so much weight. I felt as though I was losing my mind. I couldn't get anything accomplished in my life. Every minute of every day was consumed with what I was eating, or when I was going to eat again. I was so hard on myself, declaring the day an unqualified failure if I ate even a morsel of food that was supposed to be off-limits. I would string together a few good days of eating well and exercising, and then I would throw it all away over something minor, like drinking a can of Mountain Dew while at work on a stressful day. That one twelve-ounce soda would lead me to eat a large pepperoni and sausage pizza or two, foot-long cheese and meatball subs. When I was thinking logically, I knew one can of soda wasn't that bad in the grand scheme of things. But logical thinking was a rare occurrence in that state of mind. Perhaps I was just looking for an excuse to binge eat. And those excuses were quite easy to come by.

I withdrew from my family, avoiding gatherings for special occasions because I couldn't stand to see the looks on their faces, disappointed as they realized I was as heavy as ever. I remember one Christmas, before I had kids and couldn't shirk family duties, actually being ecstatic because Michael had to work the holiday. It allowed me to spend the day at home, alone, instead of being forced to attend another family event. I spent Christmas all by myself, hiding from the world and eating whatever I wanted. I was really happy and relieved, and that's what ultimately scared me the most. Who is happy when she spends the holidays alone? Someone who is not well, I was sure.

I wasn't able to avoid all family gatherings, and such was the case with that family beach trip in 2002, the one that started with such good intentions but evolved into me sneaking out at night to make a McDonald's run. Seven whole days of facing my in-laws, with a backdrop of sand and surf, bathing suits and suntan lotion. Could I be more miserable? I didn't think so, although the gods did smile upon me somewhat: It rained almost every single day, severely limiting our time by the ocean. Let me tell you: Rain at the beach is a fat girl's friend!

There was at least one sunny day, and it was the day I reached a critical point, personally. We'd spent all morning at the beach, watching our nieces and nephew dance in the surf. I tried to tell myself I didn't stand out in the crowd at all, dressed in my black T-shirt (black at the beach!) and longish khaki cropped pants (long pants! at the beach!). I was relieved when someone suggested we pack up and head back to the bungalows to fix lunch. I was loaded down, carrying a beach umbrella on a pole in one hand and a folded-up beach chair in the other (a chair that, by the way, I refused to sit on because I was afraid it would collapse under me). My butt was numb, having spent the whole morning sitting on a towel on the hard sand. We had a long way back to the cottage, and the sand was deep, my steps quite heavy. I was sweating like a pig, beads of perspiration flowing down my spine like a river. Even though I'd started out in the lead, every single family member passed me as my steps grew slower and slower.

Eventually I reached the steep staircase that led back up to street level. Taking a deep breath I started the slow journey, carrying more than three hundred pounds of flesh and various unused items of beach paraphernalia. I slowly trudged up the wooden slats, and when I finally reached the top, I made an abrupt stop. The bright sunlight started to dim, as though a huge rain cloud was passing through. But this was a cloudless day, and I knew something was wrong. I tried to steady my breath, and found that I had very little to work with. The sky above me started to spin a little, and I opened my mouth to call out to my group. Michael had already reached and crossed the street—I could see him walking way ahead with his brother, swinging our niece's hand. All of their backs were to me: my mother and father-in-law, Michael's grandmother, Michael's sister, and her kids. I tried to call to them, but no sound came out of my mouth—there was no breath to make any words. The sunlight was really dimming now, and I could feel my legs start to buckle. *Please turn around,* I thought to myself. The voice inside my head sounded as weak as I felt.

And just like that, my sister-in-law, Molly, turned back to look at me. It was a casual movement, as if she were going to ask me what I wanted for lunch, or what I'd thought of that season of *Survivor.* It was an insignificant move to her, but it meant everything to me.

My breath was back. I drew in sharply as Molly made her way toward me. "It's hot!" she exclaimed. "You okay?"

No, but I was getting there. Suddenly the sky wasn't as dim, my head wasn't as swimmy. I didn't yet trust my voice to work, so I just nodded and let her talk. I was able to get my breathing under control as we slowly walked, Molly happily chatting about her family, her kids, her life. I listened in silence, grateful for a sister-in-law who liked to talk and didn't seem to notice my lack of contribution.

We got back to the bungalow, and Michael followed me when he noticed I went straight to our bedroom. I lay on the bed and burst into tears, telling him what had happened. I also confessed the awful bingeing that had started a couple of days before. Worry clouded his face, but no anger. No judgment. Just love and concern, and it made me cry even harder.

The episode on the beach scared me into action. I didn't know exactly what had happened, but I felt it was a warning. I had to do something. The day we returned home, I called a doctor I had heard about from my coworkers, one who specifically dealt with bariatric patients. I made an appointment for the following week. I also called a therapist who had been recommended to me a couple of years earlier. I lined her up for the next week as well.

I was frightened enough to try to do something—again. Did it stop me from overeating until the appointments? No. But why would it? I knew I had a plan, that I was going to take action, so I felt I had a license to eat until then.

I had heard great things about the bariatric doctor I was going to see. It intrigued me that she was someone who devoted her practice to overweight patients—it made me feel as though my problems were legitimate and medically based. And surely she'd know what to do. This could be the answer I was looking for!

And it was. I soon learned that her weapon of choice was diet drugs. Turns out only part of fen-phen was yanked from the market; phentermine was still available, and this doctor had seen great results in her patients. I was more than a little skeptical. Did I really want to go down this road again? My feelings were still hurt from the last time, even though five or more years had passed. I just felt so cheated, so wronged. Again, I was never worried about the possible heart damage. My only concern was that losing the drugs stopped my weight loss dead in its tracks—and eventually I'd gained it all back.

My other worry was whether or not it would be effective. I'd had such great success with the combination of drugs, would just one of them do the trick? And how did I know this medication wouldn't soon be taken off the shelves as well?

The doctor explained that phentermine worked as the appetite suppressant, and she thought that was ideal for my problem. I couldn't really argue with that—it seemed to me that if you took away the overwhelming hunger, you took away most of my issues. Plus, the doctor said, in order for her to prescribe the drug to me, I would have to commit to seeing her every two weeks so that she could monitor my blood pressure and other vitals. She would perform an EKG before giving me the pills, just to make sure my heart was fine. And she would quiz me extensively about my eating and exercising plans. Taking this medicine was not a long-term solution, she stressed. I was going to have to develop habits that would take me through the rest of my life. It would not be easy, but she felt I would find success.

Really, what alternative did I have? Nothing else was working, and besides, I liked the things she proposed. Eating plan? Exercise plan? Regular check-ins with her in which I would be held accountable? I loved plans! I loved goals and charts and appointments. Since I was obsessing about it all the time anyway, this was perfect!

I enthusiastically signed up, and then almost immediately suffered from sticker shock. I knew the pills would not be covered by insurance—I'd learned that during my fen-phen days. And man, were they expensive! Seventy-five dollars a month. Plus my doctor wanted me to try Xenical, a drug designed to remove fat from food before its digested. Some people experienced pretty nasty side effects (read: accidents!), but I was game. Even on my best diet days, I still had plenty of fat in my diet. I figured this drug could only help. But again, Xenical was not covered by insurance. Another seventy dollars a month! Not to mention the doctor's visits every two weeks, which, you guess it, were not covered. Another two hundred dollars a month!

I'll never understand the rationale of insurance companies. Most will not pay for you to see a nutritionist, to join a gym, or to take an appetite suppressant. But they will pay tens of thousands of dollars for weight-loss surgery. In fact that's the only weight-loss tool they will pay for. Does that make any sense? No wonder so many people are turning to that alternative—it truly is their only (affordable) option!

The cost was rough, but I figured I had to do it. Michael and I were both working, and we didn't have kids at the time, so I felt we could make the financials work. Thankfully the weekly visits to the therapist *were* covered by insurance, and my first visit to her occurred before I started taking the diet pills.

I had been down this road before. As a teenager I'd suffered a pretty major breakdown and my parents, at my request, placed me in a mental health treatment center. I was so tired of fighting the abusive boyfriend and so sick of feeling helpless to do anything about it. I figured taking such drastic measures would be a major step toward curing me. Only, it wasn't. I checked in on a Friday and didn't see a doctor the entire weekend. I was told I would start seeing a therapist on Monday, but by that time I'd talked myself out of the need for inpatient care. Truth be told, I missed the boyfriend so much, I was already over the whole idea. So I convinced my mom to check me out, and I never went back. Thousands of dollars in bills and the legacy of having entered a mental facility, and nothing to show for it.

As I became an adult, I had a few appointments here and there with therapists, always a part of my latest plan to "get well" and "fix my problems." I never made it past the first meeting with these folks, though, because they almost immediately brought up the possibility of antidepressants. How could they know I needed something like that before they even knew me? I wasn't opposed to medication, really; I just felt that we should do some exploring first and if we reached that conclusion, then okay. I was turned off by the fact that they were suggested right off the bat, and I subsequently didn't go back to the counselors who were offering them.

I was a little less incensed when my medical doctors suggested antidepressants over the years. At least they knew me and had a great deal of information about what my problems were doing to me physically. I even agreed when my ob-gyn suggested I try a particular drug. She explained that it was used to treat mild forms of depression and one of the side effects was weight loss. Sounded like a win-win to me! I still wasn't crazy about the notion, but I agreed to try. Five days into taking the pills, Michael demanded that I cease and desist. I cried nonstop. I couldn't even function. Maybe I should have given the drugs more time. Perhaps I should have consulted with my doctor about the dosage. But I didn't, and that was my one and only experience with antidepressant medication.

I hadn't had the best of luck with mental health professionals. But for some reason I was optimistic about this latest appointment. Maybe it was because I knew I was getting medical help, and I just figured therapy would be icing on the cake. Whatever it was, I went into that meeting with a positive outlook—and I wasn't disappointed. The therapist acted genuinely interested in me and helping me find a solution. She asked great questions, and from her follow-ups, I could tell she was truly listening. And she never once mentioned antidepressants. I was feeling good about the prospects.

When I finally got the phentermine, I was ready for action. The night before, I ate to my heart's content: three plates of spaghetti, topped high with meat sauce, and garlic bread. Chocolate ice cream for dessert. And tons of Mountain Dew. I knew the next day would mark a new era, so I figured I better get it in while I could. Some crazy ways of thinking never change.

I ate a big breakfast and waited a couple of hours before taking the phentermine, when I arrived at work. In about fifteen minutes, I knew I would be just fine. The pill put me on such a high, I was knocked out, but in a good way. I found myself smiling uncontrollably, despite myself, as though I had some sort of secret. I called Michael and told him I felt GRRRREAT! And I didn't eat a thing for the rest of the day. It was glorious!

This was a new experience for me. Each day I felt my mood alter when I took my medication. It sort of "evened me out"—I just felt steady all day long. The stress of my job didn't affect me as much, and because my eating was in control, I felt more than fine. It wasn't long before some of the weight came off and people began to notice. I was getting compliments, and I was feeling in control. Life, once again, felt good. I was full of promise.

After several months on this new regimen, I'd lost sixty-five pounds. Again, I felt as though the drugs were my saving grace, exactly what I needed to get going with my weight loss. When I went to see my ob-gyn for my annual checkup, she was thrilled to see I'd lost weight, and she asked how I'd done it. I happily told her I was seeing a weight doctor who put me on phentermine. She stopped short, looking at me with a cocked head. "Is that working for you?" she asked, somewhat skeptically. Obviously, yes—the scales didn't lie! I explained to her that I felt in control, my moods were great, and I was no longer obsessed with hunger all the time. She nodded thoughtfully but didn't really have much to say. I could tell she was a bit wary. I was puzzled, but I didn't press it.

What I did want to talk to her about was getting pregnant. I was approaching thirty, and I felt as though time was running out. Michael and I would soon celebrate our tenth wedding anniversary, and our families were starting to wonder if we would ever have kids. At my heaviest, I was told I probably couldn't get pregnant, that a morbidly obese woman rarely ovulates. Now that I was losing weight, my mind inevitably turned to when I would be able to have children.

I expected this doctor to say once I completed my weight loss, I should be good to go to get pregnant. But she didn't. She asked me why I was waiting. "I've seen women much heavier than you have perfectly healthy babies," she said. "Why would you deprive yourself?"

This floored me. It went against what every other doctor had told me. Yes, I'd lost sixty-five pounds, but I still had a long, long way to go before I was considered healthy. Didn't I need to finish that mission first?

But then the other side of the argument started to make sense: How long would it take for me to lose all the weight? Another year? I wasn't getting any younger, and besides, why would I want to lose all of my weight just to turn around and gain a bunch with a pregnancy?

I so wanted to have a baby; I had wanted to be a mother almost from the moment I'd married Michael. I felt more than ready, and I knew Michael would make a terrific father. He was scared to death even at the thought, but he allowed me to take the lead on this one. I figured I would go ahead and stop birth control pills, thinking it would take several months to get pregnant. In the meantime I could still continue the medication and continue with my weight loss. You know where this is going.

Yep. First try.

And so that ended my second round of diet drugs. Lots of success, only to be stopped abruptly before I was finished losing the weight. This time, though, I had only myself to blame.

My pregnancy also stopped my going to therapy. Even though it was going well, I viewed having to visit a shrink in direct correlation with needing to lose weight. Since I was no longer trying to shed pounds, I reasoned that I could put therapy on hold. I promised myself I would go back once I gave birth and started back on track to getting healthier.

I had a beautiful baby girl and didn't gain a whole lot of weight. When Emma turned one, I was pregnant with her brother. After I had Eli, the twelve-pound newborn who suffered because I couldn't get my eating under control, I knew I was done having children and ready to finally put the weight battle to rest. My health was starting to be a major concern, and I now had two small children to consider.

This time I didn't waste efforts on other plans. I went to my new ob-gyn and asked for phentermine. She was a little wary, saying in her experience it wasn't that effective, and she wondered about the long-term risks. I convinced her that I'd done really well with it, and that I was desperate for something, anything, to work. I was more than three hundred pounds, and once again found myself at that hopeless stage. The doctor gave me a month's prescription, saying she had to see me in four weeks. I'd better show progress, she warned, or I wouldn't get the pills again from her. Relieved, I filled the script and readied to take it the next day—which of course means I ate my brains out that night!

That old, euphoric feeling came back as soon as I took the pill the next morning, and again, all felt right with the world. Once more I was struck at the mood-stabilizing effect the drug had on me, and it made me wonder if I did indeed need some sort of antidepressant. It just kind of took the edge off. After taking the medication for about two weeks, though, I noticed it wasn't lasting me all day like it used to. I at first brushed it off, thinking I was imagining things, but I secretly began to wonder if the medication was losing its effect. Still, I lost twelve pounds that first month, and my doctor was thrilled, praising my success. She happily wrote me a new prescription and told me to be back in a month.

One week into the new prescription, it was undeniable: The pills weren't working. I'd have a couple of hours of good feeling/no hunger, but then that wore off, and I was starving. Without much resistance I would binge eat, justifying my over-eating by vowing to change the way I took the medication the next day. Surely I could adjust it and do better, right? I played this game for the rest of the month, torturing myself daily with should-I-or-should-I-not-eat arguments that always landed me at the drive-thru. I wound up gaining back five pounds.

My doctor nodded patiently as I explained (lied) to her that it had been a tough month. I told her I forgot to take my medicine a lot, and I was sure it would work again once I got my act together. She showed no emotion whatsoever as she told me she was not giving me a new prescription and that I would have to get my act together on my own. I tried not to look so desperate, but I dissolved into tears. She seemed pretty unmoved, and I felt as though I'd been punched in the gut.

I was still smarting a couple of days later when her nurse called and suggested I find a general practitioner. It seemed this doctor only wanted to see me for ob-gyn issues. I cried even more, but I was also mad. Who the hell did she think she was? In my mind, she had such a God complex. "No! You can't have it!" I imagined her saying cruelly, yanking away my one shot at losing weight.

If I'm being honest, I can't really blame her. She'd warned me she wasn't a huge fan of the drug, and that I would have to play by the rules. I hadn't, so she stopped playing. But where did that leave me? I felt as though she'd abandoned me and I had nowhere to turn.

The nurse suggested a general practitioner, and I made an appointment. Maybe this doctor would give me a script for phentermine—maybe if I explained everything, she would understand! Clearly I was deluding myself. The medication had stopped working, but I still thought there was hope, that the only way I was going to lose weight was with that kind of help. As I waited to see the new doctor, I gave myself a pep talk. *Don't be too anxious,* I told myself. *Play it cool. Let her come to the conclusion so it won't look like that's what you're shopping for.*

The doctor seemed perfectly nice. I explained to her my history, how I'd gained the weight after I'd gotten married, and how I had tried any number of ways to lose it over the years, with minimal success. I almost couldn't believe it when I started really opening up. I tearfully told her that sometimes I felt like I was losing my mind, that all I thought about was how to stop eating, stop abusing food. I felt stuck in an endless cycle—with no way out—and I was helpless. She seemed to really listen, really hear what I was saying. She made it easy to be honest about my feelings.

When I'd finished, she expressed her sympathy and concern. She said she wanted to go get something for me off her desk, and she excused herself. I dried my tears and waited for her to return, feeling really hopeful for the first time in quite a while. This doctor was going to hear me. She really got what I was trying to say.

The doctor came back in with papers in her hand. "I printed for you a copy of the Food Pyramid," she started. My jaw dropped to the floor as she continued. "I want you to see what your goals should be in terms of what kinds of food you should be eating."

I almost expected her to burst out in laughter and say, "Just kidding!" But as she droned on and on about the importance of a balanced diet, I slowly began to realize just how serious she was. And I was angry. I was seething. Hot, angry tears seared my vision. My heart pounded so loudly in my chest, I was sure she could hear it.

Was she insane? Had my words meant nothing to her? I had poured my heart out to this woman, admitting that I thought I was addicted to food and that I might be a little crazy. Her answer was for me to look at the Food Pyramid and try to eat a more balanced diet?! *Seriously?*

But wait, she wasn't finished. "I also think you should look into this faith-based organization. It's called TOPS, or Taking Off Pounds Sensibly. They have several meeting locations in this area. I found one within a couple of miles of your zip code."

She handed me the sheet. She had made an effort, although a horribly stupid one. I couldn't criticize her intentions, I supposed. But I also couldn't believe that a medical doctor couldn't see what a real mess of a person she had before her, and how could she possibly think my answer was the Food Pyramid and a church support group? Was she an idiot?

I swallowed hard, trying my best to restrain my emotions. I was mad, but I wasn't about to give up on what I thought was my only hope. "Thanks for this," I said softly. "I was wondering . . . what do you think about phentermine? The few times I've had success, it was because of medication," I said, rather weakly.

She nodded. "Well, I think it's definitely an option for us," she started, and my heart immediately lifted. Maybe she wasn't so bad! Maybe she wasn't so clueless!

"But," she said, "I would have to see you successfully complete a three-month plan of a good diet and exercise before I could prescribe that for you."

I was sure I hadn't heard correctly. I indicated so, but she repeated the same thing. If I was floored before, I was absolutely flabbergasted now. Three months? I couldn't even put three days together! Why in the world did she think I was there? Why was I seeking her help if I could do it on my own?

It became real clear, real quick that this doctor wasn't going to help me, and I was incredibly sad. How could she not understand? How could no one understand what I was going through? And if that was the case, how was I ever going to solve the problem?

I knew there wasn't much research about how phentermine affects the body. I knew that the whole fen-phen fiasco had made doctors skittish. But really, what's the alternative? Walk around with an extra two hundred pounds, letting it wreak havoc on my heart? I had diabetes and high blood pressure— I was marching toward an early grave. If I knew something worked—something would help me get the weight off—didn't it make sense to do it, whatever the cost?

That same argument would come up in the not-so-distant future.

For right then I decided to try one more doctor. My husband had a general practitioner whom I'd seen for minor things and who'd invited me to become a regular patient. I gave myself the same pep talk while I waited in his waiting room: *Play it cool, Jennifer. Don't be too anxious.* As I sat on the exam table, I calmly told him about all my efforts to lose weight, mostly to no avail. And then I laid my cards right on the table: "I've had the most success when I've taken phentermine, and I'd like to try it again," I said firmly.

This doctor, a man, was busy writing notes in my chart, and he didn't look up when I stopped talking. "I'm not sure those are effective," he said, still writing.

"Why not?" I shot back before I could help myself.

This time, he looked up at me.

My face felt hot, and I looked away. "I mean, nothing else is working and I am desperate here. I'll try anything, just please." I met his glance again, sure that I had pleading in my eyes.

He nodded. "Yes, we can try it," he said casually.

No lectures, no God-like stance, no threats. He gave me the medicine. I could have kissed him.

I was determined not to waste this go-around. I didn't know if I'd get the chance again. I took the medicine enthusiastically. I got the familiar buzz right off, and I was so happy. I was on my way.

The hunger punched through before lunchtime.

It was over. The medicine didn't work anymore.

What in the hell was I going to do now?

7

Sex and the Fat Girl

DECEMBER 31, 2006

I'm hiding again. This time I'm not sneaking around in order to eat (although let's face it—that is sure to come later). No, this time I am hiding from my husband. Michael wants sex. He's been dropping hints all day: an extra long hug from behind as I wash dishes at the sink, a whistle and a grin as I walk by with a load of laundry. After thirteen years of marriage, I know the signs, and my husband is letting me know that today is the day. He will wait no more. He must have me now.

Every time I think about it, my stomach turns in knots so big I can't breathe. My skin crawls, like ants setting my flesh on fire. I want to cry, but my sobs stick in my throat.

I should be dropping to my knees, thanking God profusely for giving me such an unbelievably wonderful husband. Why he didn't leave long ago, when the weight began to pile on and my psychosis really started to fester, I will never understand. Any other man would have run for the hills. Not only is the weight gain a physical turnoff, but the accompanying behavior is also unbearable. Mood swings, crying jags, defensiveness up the wazoo. And the lies! Lying about what I'm eating, where I'm going, how I've spent our money. How could he remain by my side when I am pushing him away with all my might?

But stay he does. And he still wants me. This I will never, ever be capable of comprehending. I weigh more than three hundred pounds. I am revolting. My body is a disfigured mess. I am covered in stretch marks—some a silvery, translucent color, others bright purple and rough to the touch. My swollen belly has so many layers, you could lose small appliances in it. My breasts, never anything to brag about in the first place, are now unrecognizable blobs that hang due south. I haven't seen my vagina in years. I assume it's still there, but I have no first-hand account of its existence, let alone its appearance. My skin is scaly, my hair is ratty and thinning, and I have questionable body odors.

Yeah. I'm a lover boy's dream.

When he touches me, I can't sit still. I want to jump out of my skin. I change the subject. I create an emergency that I must tend to right away, anything to get away from being held. How can Michael not do the same? How can he desire me? Is his love that blind?

Or is he pretending for me? Yes, that must be it. How could it be anything else? There is no way he wants to make love to such a horrible beast of a woman—no way he could choose to be with me—if it weren't for his sense of duty, of obligation. He's taking pity on me. He's honoring our marriage vows, even though he must want desperately to find the out clause. We have children, after all; he can't leave now. He's too much of a stand-up guy for that. And I do believe he loves me, based on what we used to be. He's making the most of a bad situation, I suppose. He is still a man. He still has needs. And I am his wife—I should meet those needs. I should *want* to meet those needs.

But every touch reminds me of what I have become. When he tries, and fails, to wrap his arms around me, I think of what an odd-shaped pair we make: I am more than twice his size. That's not right! It isn't natural! I am supposed to be the dainty wife, the little woman. Sadly, I'd have to date Goliath in order to fit that description.

When I'm with him, I can't concentrate on my love for him or on trying to rekindle that physical desire. All I can do is wallow in self-pity, wondering how I allowed this to happen. Images of what our physical relationship used to be engulf me, and I push away even harder. I know those days are gone because I can't get a grip.

I have ruined us.

He's still here. So finally, when I can't avoid it any longer, we have sex. About once a month I grit my teeth and force myself to go through with it. It's like facing a firing squad. I try to pretend to like it, and sometimes for a little bit I manage to fool myself. When he kisses me, I faintly recall the burning desire that enveloped us in the early days of our relationship. We were insatiable. We made love anytime, anywhere, all the time. Because I knew how much he loved me, I was confident and uninhibited, and our sex life was as active and as satisfying as it could be. Now I close my eyes and try to think of that time, and I momentarily get lost in the memory of what we once were. I return Michael's passionate kiss and, for that brief moment, I can't wait to consummate our love once more.

And then, like a bolt of lightning slamming into the summer sky, I remember the cold, hard reality of my situation. I can't make love the old-fashioned way. My self-consciousness takes over, and I won't allow my husband to climb on top of me. My big belly is too much of a distraction; I'm way too ashamed to allow it to come between us. I stop Michael so that we can reposition ourselves. He reluctantly complies, and remorse and regret threaten to pull me under yet again. Good thing I'm not facing him. Even in the pitch-dark bedroom, he would detect the tears that have sprung to my eyes. If he were allowed to hold me properly, he would know the grief I feel. *It's better this way,* I tell myself. *Better for all involved.*

For the last ten years, we've had sex in only one position. I won't be so crass as to come out and say which one that is; you can probably figure it out. It's the one where my huge stomach is the least obtrusive.

Our intimacy suffers. There's no kissing, no stroking of each other's faces, no holding him in my arms. It's a purely mechanical move, a physical means to an end. Yes, the outcome for both of us is a biological victory. Climax is achieved, usually on both sides. But I miss the closeness that used to accompany our passion, the togetherness we felt alongside the physical pleasure. The minute, no the second, it's over, I'm racked with silent sobs. I feel so guilty for allowing this to happen to our marriage. I am solely responsible, and it is devastating.

What kind of woman am I? I binge eat, stuffing myself with so much food that I am sick. I don't try hard enough to find clothes that fit me, and look like a royal mess most of the time. And I can't maintain a proper physical relationship with my husband. I am a failure in every sense of the word. I try to do something about these things; each day dawns with a new plan for me to take control, trying to implement ways to get back to the woman I once was. But I always fail, doomed to suffer in this seemingly self-imposed exile for what feels like eternity. I am trapped, and I am suffocating.

⟋⟍

Love is supposed to hurt. That's what I have always believed, no matter how hard Michael has tried to change that for me. Growing up, I didn't have the greatest example of how men are supposed to treat women, what girls should expect from boys. My dad, while not outright abusive to my mom, was an absent husband. He worked hard and provided for his family, but he fought his own demons and they kept him away from us most of the time. He drank heavily and would "go to bed" early in the evening, which I would later learn meant he would pass out in his room. He never took Mom out, never maintained a social life with her as a couple. She hardly ever took vacations; she rarely attended events with friends. She was ashamed to show up without a husband, so she simply didn't attend. He wallowed in whatever drove him to self-destruct, and she paid the price, year after year. Boy, does this sound familiar.

My dad never treated me unkindly. He always picked me up from school when he was supposed to, and he provided for any need or want that I had, whether it was clothes for school or a new bike for my birthday, even a car when I turned sixteen. But he was, for the most part, emotionally absent as a father. I knew that he loved me, although he rarely said so. He grew up with parents who showed virtually no affection, and so he never felt comfortable doing so himself. I remember one time telling my mother that I didn't know if my dad loved me because he never told me. The next morning, there was an awkward silence as he drove me to school. You could tell he was trying to find a way to say something but was having great difficulty. When the car stopped, he looked down at his hands and very softly said, "I love you." Even at such a young age, I could tell how hard it was for him to say it, and it meant so much to me, I have never forgotten. A couple of years later, I was leaving to spend two weeks with my cousin in Virginia Beach. My dad had to leave for work before I got up, and he wouldn't see me before I left. There was a note from him on the kitchen table, in his gorgeous handwritten script. He told me to be safe and to have a good time. And he wrote, "I love you." I saved that little piece of ruled notebook paper for years, finally losing it when I went away to college. I was devastated when I couldn't find it; that note meant the world to me.

I loved my father with all my heart, and we did have a closer relationship when I became an adult. He died several years ago, and I miss him every day. But if a young girl learns how to expect a man to treat her from how her father treats her, then I was sorely lacking. Yes, he loved me and provided for me, but I had to work so hard to get even a scrap of real demonstration of that love. I was constantly trying to wring it out of him, impress him enough so that he would be bowled over by me. I was too young to understand that he gave me all that he could, that he was incapable of showing me how much he cared. All I knew was that he never told me I was pretty, never acted as though he thought I was very smart or very good at much of anything. He never shared any of my interests—or pretended to—as most parents are forced to do from time to time. I was his daughter, and for that he loved me, but there was nothing about me that terribly impressed him. That's what I took from growing up, and it was devastating for my self-esteem.

What didn't help was that I had two older brothers who *did* have my father's attention. My father loved sports and my brothers excelled in sports, so they bonded endlessly over baseball and basketball. I sucked at sports. I had no coordination and no real desire to try and learn. While I was being dragged to every youth athletic event in the state, you would find me on the bleachers with my nose in a book. My dad could not relate to this, and that was a fatal flaw in our relationship. I would watch him connect with my brothers, and I would feel hurt and confused. Why couldn't he talk to me like that? I was always trying to get his attention, connect with him with one thing or another, but it never worked. Once, I remember him taking me and my brothers to a store and letting us pick out whatever we wanted. I felt giddy riding in the car, not only from the pending purchase, but from being included with the boys, spending some bonding time with my dad. I picked out a baby doll that drank a bottle and wet her diaper. My brothers picked out a basketball goal. We went home and my dad and brothers spent the rest of the afternoon in the backyard, building the goal and putting it into the ground. I stayed in my room and played with my doll, alone. My window overlooked the backyard, and I could see them working together, laughing, and then playing once they were finished. I felt like a complete outsider.

If I thought my relationship with my father was somewhat lacking, my relationship with my brothers was downright destructive. They were mean, and they were cruel. They admit that now, although they question if it was quite as bad as I make it out to be. It was. We were never, ever close, and I really don't know why. My mom grew up with four brothers, and she says when she saw my brothers tease me, she chalked it up to normal sibling rivalry. It was not normal. They called me "fat bitch" on a daily basis, probably from the age of eight. I was hit and punched quite regularly, by two older brothers who were always bigger and stronger and who often ganged up on me. They made a sport of embarrassing me in front of others, whether it was to call me names in front of their friends or physically attack me in front of mine. Yes, I called them names. Yes, I tried to hit them back. But I was outnumbered and out-powered. They called me ugly, fat, smelly, bitch, dumbass—you name it. I heard every insult imaginable and then some.

As adults we have somewhat mended fences; I'm closer to one brother than I am to the other. When my niece was about nine years old, she came to me at a Thanksgiving gathering, her eyes big and brown and brimming with tears. She said her grandmother, my mother, had given her one of my books from when I was little. In the back she found a message written in pencil: "Jennifer is a big, fat roach!" She tearfully told me that she asked her dad who wrote that and he admitted he had, and he deeply regretted it. As I wiped her tears and told her I was okay, I wondered if I ever would be.

When it came time for me to become interested in boys, I had the following knowledge: My father, though never cruel, had never once told me I had anything of value to offer—that I was pretty or smart or possessed any other redeeming quality that the male species would find attractive. And I had two brothers who never missed an opportunity to tell me I was fat, ugly, disgusting, repulsive, and dumb.

What kind of men do you think I hoped to attract?

When I was fourteen I became involved with a seventeen-year-old who was emotionally absent and pretty indifferent to my existence. This, unfortunately, didn't deter me. I was used to this; this was normal. Why would I expect more, why would I think I deserved better? No one ever told me or showed me that. No, I became convinced that my fate was to turn this boy around, convince him that he loved me, that he wanted me, and that I was enough for him. I was forever trying to impress him, to win him over. It's so obvious to me now what I was doing—trying to re-create my failed relationships with my father and brothers, but with a happier, more successful conclusion.

Of course it didn't work. This boy, much like my father and my brothers, couldn't be changed, at least not by me. I spent five years with him, and the damage took my already fragile self-esteem and pulverized it beyond recognition. He used me, cheated on me, and rarely acknowledged me in public as his girl-friend. He also had a very hard time showing affection, and he rarely gave me compliments or told me I was in any way impor-tant to him. I knew he treated me poorly, and I knew about the other girls. I didn't like it, of course; I fought him, cried, begged, and threatened to leave him constantly. I always came back, though, after every public embarrassment, every humiliation. I thought if I tried harder—if I bought him things, if I lost weight and looked better—I would finally be enough for him, I would win him over for good. Of course that didn't happen.

It's so easy to look at this situation from the outside and say, *Why didn't I just leave him? Why did I put up with someone who clearly didn't want me?* When I was thinking rationally, I would ask these things of myself. But most of my thinking was not rational. I generally thought that I couldn't do any better, that this was the kind of man I was destined to have and it was my lot in life to make the best of it. Every night I would cry over a missed phone call or a forgotten date, begging God to please get me out of this nightmare. But the next morning would come and I would have thought of a new plan to try to win him over, to get him to realize I was the one for him. It was the same destructive pattern I would later use when it came to my weight.

I knew what a god-awful situation I was in. My parents were furious and demanded that I end the relationship. I couldn't. My friends, tired of hearing me cry for years and years, told me I had to dump him or I would lose them. I wouldn't end it; I felt like I couldn't live without him. I lost friendships. I knew it was wrong, but I felt powerless to stop it. It was a situation I wanted to end, most of the time, but I felt too weak to let it go.

That New Year's Eve in 1990, when my bingeing was born, was all an effort to finally convince him that I was worth loving. I had had enough. I broke it off with him, and I managed to stay away for a few months. I lost weight and looked great. He heard about it and sought me out, saying all the right things to get me back. Of course I went back—he was the reason I'd lost the weight in the first place. But I was surprised when he started trying to get me to eat more. He never came out and said it, but I figured out he didn't like the fact that I had lost weight. I think it threatened him and the hold he had over me; suddenly he realized I could be attractive to others. Does this sound like a man who loved, cared for, and wanted the best for me?

I was still in this destructive relationship when I went away to college. I thought the distance would make our relationship stronger, that he would realize I had other things going for me and he better get smart and appreciate what he had. What I didn't count on was meeting the man of my dreams—and having him like me, too.

Michael had a girlfriend, and I had a boyfriend. But that didn't stop us from finding each other. When he showed interest in me, I literally couldn't believe it. He was cute, smart, funny . . . and he was really, really nice. How could he like me? What was the catch? I was head over heels for him, but I knew he was involved with someone else. He was clearly torn: He liked me and wanted to be with me, but he had been with her for a long time and felt obligated to her. Their relationship was not a good one, but he didn't want to hurt her; he never wanted to hurt anybody. I (stupidly) told him that if he wanted to stay with her and still see me, I would understand and do whatever he wanted. This really speaks to my low self-esteem and what I thought I was worth. I just assumed that no man would find me worthy of a sacrifice. Thank God Michael wasn't the kind of man to take advantage of a girl who didn't think much of herself. He broke it off with his girlfriend and pledged his love for me. I was over the moon, but I still couldn't believe it. He did that for me? He wanted to be with me, just me?

Needless to say I kicked my destructive boyfriend to the curb. I had to laugh to myself at how hurt he was when I told him I had found someone else and that I was leaving him. It was like he chose that moment to realize I was a good catch. Talk about too little, too late. I marveled at how easy it was for me to say good-bye to him after all those years of hurt and struggle. I viewed it as Michael saving me from that bad situation; he was the one to give me the strength that I had needed for so long.

I never gave myself any credit for ending the relationship. On the contrary, I viewed myself as weak and unable to help myself. It was only after Michael loved me that I found the strength to cut the abusive boyfriend out of my life. This warped way of thinking would repeat itself later in my life.

To say I was on cloud nine with Michael is a huge understatement. I finally had what I had been seeking for so long: a man who truly loved me and cared about me. And he was quite demonstrative of that love. He called me "pretty" several times a day, and I blushed profusely. He constantly stroked my face or put his arm around me. I loved the affection, but I had a really hard time with it—I wasn't used to someone showing me how much I mattered to them. I craved the attention, but I had a hard time returning the love. I didn't really know how. I could count on one hand how many times my father had hugged me. The destructive boyfriend could be somewhat affectionate in private, but never, ever when we went out. When Michael grabbed my hand and held it as we walked across campus, I squirmed. I was embarrassed. Did he really want people to see him holding my hand? Wasn't he worried what others would think? Of course he wasn't, but that was the low opinion I had of myself. Michael recognized my struggle, and he assured me constantly that I was someone he could be proud of being with. I tried really hard to believe it.

Ours was a whirlwind romance. We were married a year and a half after we got together. He was funny, we shared the same interests, and he loved me unconditionally and unabashedly. I never, ever thought I would be so lucky.

Gone was the everyday struggle I'd had while in that abusive relationship. I had known I was in a very bad situation, but I was unable to get myself out of it. With Michael, that no longer existed, and I felt so very happy. For the first time in my life, I was constantly reminded how much I was loved.

And all of a sudden, the weight started to pile on.

I quickly gained back all the weight I'd lost in high school. At first I wasn't too worried about it; I chalked it up to my being in love and focused on Michael and not as vigilant as I should be about what I was eating and how often I exercised. But for the first time, it didn't stop there. I kept gaining weight, and as our wedding approached, I was tipping the scales at 180, bigger than I had ever been. If Michael noticed, he didn't mention it, but I could sure tell. I couldn't figure out why I was having such a hard time. I'd finally gotten the love and affection I had always so desperately wanted. Why did I feel the need to overeat?

Looking back I truly think the weight gain started as a way for me to self-destruct. There is something in my makeup that wants me to be unhappy—something inside me that is convinced I don't deserve good things in my life. Low self-esteem led me into that destructive relationship and kept me there for five years. When I finally managed to break free from that and find someone who truly loved and wanted to be with me, I had to find another way to self-sabotage. I had found true love, I was on an exciting career path, and things in my life were going swimmingly. All these good things didn't sit well with the little voice deep within me, the one that constantly reminded me I was worthless and stupid and ugly. I had to try to find a way to ruin it all. The beast started to rear its head.

Of course it took me years to see the pattern and figure out what was happening. At the time, I panicked over the sudden weight gain and tried desperately to stop it from getting worse. I failed. On our first wedding anniversary I was well over two hundred pounds, and it only grew worse from there. The giddiness I had over my relationship with Michael was replaced with a sinking, quicksand-type existence. I was desperate to stop the downslide, but powerless to make any real change stick. My career dreams were dashed, my relationships with friends and loved ones suffered, and, most devastatingly, my marriage struggled. I had fought so hard to get a man who treated me wonderfully, and all I could feel was misery. Trust issues popped up and our intimacy took a beating. And it was all my fault. Not only was I powerless to fix it, I couldn't even explain the problem. Why was I so hell-bent on ruining every good thing in my life? And would I ever be able to stop it? I never completely lost hope, but optimism was a rare and fleeting thing.

8

Skulls and Crossbones

11-16-01

Dear Mrs. Joyner:

We reviewed your application for a 30 Year Level Term II contract. After careful consideration, we regret that we cannot provide the coverage as requested and as a result, no coverage exists under the terms of this application.

Insurance companies have established underwriting practices which guide them in selecting risks according to predetermined criteria. Although these criteria vary between companies, they are all developed based on actuarial statistics and mortality experience.

Our underwriting guidelines, relating to your build, will not allow us to grant the coverage you applied for because the potential for increased mortality makes the risk greater than was anticipated in our premium rates . . .

Wow. I know things are pretty dire, but there's nothing quite like reading it in print. My initial application for life insurance has been denied because I am too fat and the chances of my dying are too great. You would think receiving a letter like this would be the a-ha moment I've been looking for, the rock-bottom place I've been trying to find for so long. My health is too much of a risk for the company to take on—I could die at any moment. I better do something right away to save my life, before I prove them right.

It's a sobering notice. I cry when I read the letter, stuffing it into my purse before Michael can see it. I'm ashamed and embarrassed. Too fat to insure? Too much of a chance that I will die prematurely? I'm twenty-nine years old! For two days I keep the news to myself, wondering how I'm going to tell my husband about this latest humiliating rejection. When the insurance agent calls, I swallow hard, waiting for him to reiterate the company's decision, but he has different news for me: They *will* offer me coverage, just at double the rate they are charging for my husband's. So . . . I am insurable? I'm not too much of a risk? I knew it! I can't be that bad! Never mind the coverage is going to be unbelievably expensive—that I will have to pay so much more than the average person my age. That doesn't matter to me at this moment. All I can focus on is that I do indeed qualify for life insurance—I have not been rejected.

⟡

At this point in my life, my weight is still mostly an issue of vanity. I hate having to scour the misses sportswear area of the department stores, hoping and praying something will actually fit. I desperately want to be an on-air reporter, and I know it will never happen unless I find some way to shed pounds. My weight makes everyday breathing harder, and it compromises my ability to perform any sort of lengthy physical activity. But I'm just not ready to consider that my very life is at risk. For me it's all about looking better—and feeling better about the way I look.

All of that will change soon enough.

In the meantime I simply nod when my doctors warn me about what my future could hold. I'm already prediabetic, meaning if I don't do something soon, I could develop the disease. I have a family history, and my weight is also a major risk factor. The doctors tell me what life is like for a person with diabetes: medication for life, possibly having to have daily insulin shots, difficulty with pregnancies. I listen and nod, and then I promptly forget what they say. I'm in my twenties, after all. I have years to worry about stuff like that. Besides, I'm not going to keep this weight on for long! My plans will finally work out and I'm going to be slim and trim in no time. No need to worry about that health stuff, I reason. The real risks are years away, and the weight will be long gone by then.

I'm not ready to consider my health with any great urgency, but I'm more than willing to pin my problems on it. The doctor I'd gone to see in 1997, the one who initially put me on fenphen, also ordered a round of tests to see if there was any medical reason for this huge weight gain. She called me a couple of weeks later—when I was in the middle of taking the diet drugs and loving the effects they were having—to tell me that my blood levels were borderline for hypothyroidism. She explained that it could be the reason for the weight gain, and for the hair loss. She wanted to send me to a specialist for further testing, but was hopeful for a diagnosis—and that would mean medication, and hopefully, some improvement in my symptoms.

I was overjoyed. *It's not my fault! This didn't happen to me because I'm lazy or gluttonous. I have a medical condition! There's a reason . . . and medicine!* I was so excited by the news, and so relieved to get what I thought was a definitive answer from a person with authority.

Of course, I was getting ahead of myself. The doctor wasn't sure, and that's why she was sending me to an endocrinologist. Still, her phone call couldn't have come at a better time. In the bathtub earlier that day, I'd noticed my first stretch mark. It was an angry crimson color, and it streaked its way down my abdomen, gnarling my skin with ragged bumps, toward my navel. It was a bright ugly reminder of what was happening to my body. I was never a fan of my naked image, and now I felt even more ashamed. I could get rid of extra pounds, but would the scars ever go away? I felt marked for life.

With much hope and anticipation, I made the appointment with the specialist, traveling more than two hours to see him the following week. His office was a two-room dump of a space, with his wife acting as both his receptionist and his nurse. I looked around skeptically as I waited. This was the answer to my prayers? More doubt crept in when I actually met him: He was no younger than eighty, with wispy, white hair standing up all over his head. He looked like a mad scientist. Still, I had a lot of respect for the doctor who recommended him, so I decided to give him a chance.

He did a brief physical exam and noted that I was starting to get "the stripes." I was confused for a moment, until I figured out that he was referring to the new stretch mark. *Great,* I thought. *I'm striped now.* He was odd in a few other ways, asking me about the water bottle I carried with me. I told him I thought drinking water would help me lose weight, and he laughed at me. Laughed at me! He said all it would help me do was go to the bathroom more.

His wife/receptionist/nurse drew blood for a new test, and I got the heck out of there. He was strange and rude, but I still hoped he could help me. You can be quirky, but still brilliant, right? A diagnosis would mean that not only would I get the medical help I needed, but also that I could possibly start to forgive myself for letting things get this bad.

The call came a week later. My blood level was normal; I did not have hypothyroidism. You would think I would have been devastated, but I wasn't. I was mad. I thought the guy was a quack, and there was no way he could be right. I had the weight gain! I had the hair loss! Of course I had hypothyroidism! I had to!

I couldn't accept what this doctor had to say, so on my own I went to see an endocrinologist at Duke University, sure that the experts there would uncover the truth. I saw a normal-looking doctor with an average-looking office, and I underwent another blood test. But the answer was the same: My blood level was normal, and I did not have hypothyroidism.

Now I was devastated. Why did I go through all of that, only to be disappointed? I had hoped to learn that I was not the lazy, undisciplined freak I was starting to convince myself I was—I had almost been ready to give myself a break. I felt like all that hope had been ripped out from under me.

What saved me from being taken under by this turn of events was the fact that I was still losing weight, thanks to the fen-phen. I could face anything as long as the scales were going in the right direction. Still—it did mark how I would treat such events in the future.

◯◯

In early 2001, after I'd stopped taking fen-phen and had gained all the weight back, the thyroid issue popped up again. This time I was heavier than I'd ever been and despondent about my inability to do anything about it. At my yearly physical my gynecologist ran a routine blood panel. I didn't even allow myself to hope for an answer—I couldn't go there. So I was truly surprised when I got the phone call from her office a few days later: My blood levels showed I clearly had hypothyroidism. No borderline results, no further testing needed. I would be starting medication right away.

I fell back onto my bed, dissolving into tears. I cried because deep down I still hadn't believed those doctors when they said my tests were normal. I had convinced myself that my problems were medical in nature. And finally, years later, I was being vindicated. But most of all I cried with relief. I was weary from the fight, and I was finally going to get some help—assistance that would not be yanked away from me without notice, a real solution that would help rid me of this problem for life. I wasn't bitter at what I considered to be a misdiagnosis for all those years; I was just grateful that the wrong had been righted and I was going to benefit. Finally I was going to be fixed.

The nurse called to tell me about the medication she'd phoned in to the pharmacy. She explained that it would take a little while to see any real changes, but I would eventually notice my energy level increase, my hair loss subside, and, yes, some weight loss. I choked back tears, thanking her profusely before heading out right away to pick up the medicine. I didn't want to waste any more time.

After taking the medication for two weeks, I didn't notice any improvement. Hair was still clogging the shower drain, my energy was almost nil, and I was just as heavy as I'd been before. I called the nurse, and she assured me that the pills would work; I just needed to give it more time. I was starting to worry a little, but I quickly brushed those concerns aside. *Don't do this to yourself, Jennifer,* I said. *This is the break you need.*

For once, let yourself off the hook. Enjoy!

Sadly, it wasn't what I'd hoped for. Two months went by, and there was no change. I went to see the doctor, and she was stumped. She agreed I should have seen an improvement by then, so she increased the dosage. I waited for signs of improvement, but they didn't come. A new blood test showed the higher dosage was too much, and the doctor had to dial back my medication. The blood work did verify that my thyroid was being helped by the medicine; the pills were working. But my symptoms were as bad as ever, and now there was no way of knowing if they would ever be helped.

I truly didn't know what I was supposed to do with this latest failure. Again all I could think of was how the medication was supposed to help me lose weight and stop the hair loss. If it wasn't doing that, then why take it? I was angry and I was bitter . . . and I stopped taking the medication. What was the point? It was just empty promises to me, and I was done.

In later years, during my pregnancies, I'd read about the importance of taking medication for hypothyroidism and how if you didn't, you could put the baby at risk. So I took the medicine religiously, every day for nine months, with both pregnancies. While the weight loss wasn't a factor, I noticed my hair loss did not improve, further convincing me that the medication wasn't doing me any good. As soon as I had the babies, I stopped taking it.

Any reasonable person would ask why I stopped the medication. Sure, there was no physical evidence it was helping me, but there also weren't any negative side effects. Why not do what my doctor asked and just take the stupid pill? I really have no explanation for this—it makes complete sense that I shouldn't go off on my own and make these decisions without any factual basis. I just didn't want to take them—having to take a pill every day made me feel like I was sick. I knew there was something wrong with me, for sure, but if I were going to have to take maintenance drugs, then I would have to see a physical benefit. Period.

In 2007, when my health was reaching a critical point, I had a doctor question me about my latest blood work. "Are you taking your Synthroid?" she asked. "Because your levels are really low."

Usually I would just make up a lame excuse, not wanting to admit to a doctor some of my rogue ways of thinking. But this time I was full-on depressed, and just jaded at the whole medical community. "No, I don't take it," I said bluntly. "It doesn't do me any good."

She looked baffled. "You know, I don't think I've ever had to convince someone to take their thyroid medication. Usually women are thrilled to hear there's a problem and a solution."

I snorted. Been there, done that. I had tons of problems, and I was starting to be convinced there was no cure.

Health was hardly ever my focus. And when it was, I was usually disappointed in the outcome, as with the whole thyroid situation. I just wanted things to be black-and-white—if there was a problem, I wanted a cure. Period. No gray areas. No let's try this, let's see if that works. I guess I didn't have patience for any of it, which is pretty ridiculous, seeing how I'd been morbidly obese for years. Why hadn't I lost patience with that? Stubbornly, I dwelled on all the emotional issues, as well as the problems with my appearance, that my weight gain had brought on, and I did not devote enough time to the toll it was taking on my physical well-being.

That slowly started to change once I had children. And it didn't change by choice, but out of necessity: For me, being pregnant meant I could no longer ignore my physical problems.

༐

When I first found out we were having a baby, I was ecstatic. Michael and I had waited for so long, watched so many friends and family members become parents, welcoming new additions. Finally it was our turn. Sure, I would have liked to be thinner; as it was, I was still very heavy when I became pregnant with my daughter, Emma. But I had just lost a lot of weight, and I was in a pretty good place emotionally. I was coming off the daily torture that is binge eating, and I was starting to have more natural, realistic thoughts when it came to what went into my mouth. Yes, I still ate too much, and too many of the wrong foods, but hey! I was pregnant! I was with child. That's license, right? For the first time in really my whole life, I ate without guilt. I didn't beat myself up with every indulgence, and that was so liberating. I could go through my days feeling good about myself and my situation, something that was so rare for me, I hardly knew what to do with it. And because I was in a good place, because I gave myself a break, I didn't binge. I never once overstuffed myself with food, making frantic promises to do better the next day. I didn't have to live under that threat umbrella. I was free.

All of that soon came to a screeching halt.

On the day I went in for my glucose test, where they determine if you're suffering from gestational diabetes, I clearly had no clue. I'd been at work all day and thought the hour-long drive to the doctor's office was the perfect time to drink a nice cold twenty-ounce bottle of Mountain Dew. Um . . . hello? Blood glucose test? Sugar? Probably not a good idea! Still, it wasn't like they told me to fast or anything, and I figured I should go about my normal routine. I was still drinking one soda a day, and I didn't think much about it.

I flunked the test.

It was only then that I truly considered the possibility of diabetes. Sure, this was gestational diabetes, a condition that would likely go away once my pregnancy was complete. But until then I would have to do all kinds of special things to monitor my health and that of my baby. Plus, having gestational diabetes makes you more prone to develop the disease later in life.

I was devastated. Gone was the liberating feeling I'd had about eating; now I would have to worry over every little thing that went into my mouth. I'd have to monitor my blood sugar levels by sticking myself with a needle every day. And I would agonize about my unborn baby's health.

Not how I envisioned my pregnancy.

I had a really hard time following the diet plan. My limited palate made it hard for me to find good foods to eat—ones that I actually liked. On a good day I was a carb-obsessed freak: breads, chips, sodas, and so on. And we already know how I felt about sugar—it deserved its own level on my personal food pyramid. This diet, however, called for no sugar and low carbs. For a person who'd gained more than 150 pounds because she couldn't control her urges to overeat, and to eat the wrong foods, it was quite a lot to ask. How was I ever going to do this?

Slowly, believe it or not, I made progress. I learned to eat hamburgers without buns. I skipped the fries and (most of) the sodas, opting instead to snack on nuts and cheese and to drink water. Of course I found ways to cheat. I promised myself that if I was good all week, I could have whatever I wanted for dinner on Saturday, for example. I also got the hang of using the needle to check my blood sugar, and I learned to use that to my eating advantage. I kept a food diary and learned what foods made my blood sugar rise and what foods I could get away with eating. I found that if I simply scraped the toppings off of a piece of pizza without eating the crust, I was fine—or if I waited until the early evening to give in to my craving for soda, my blood sugar wasn't so bad. I was very disciplined about find-ing what worked, and it paid off. My doctor was pleased with my sugar levels and with the baby's growth. My fear began to subside, and I found an inner peace with doing what was best for my baby.

Looking back, I am proud that I was able to step up for Emma's sake. I'd always hoped somewhere deep within me, willpower did in fact exist, and here I had some proof. But I'm a little sad that it took pregnancy for me to have the strength to finally do what was necessary. I thought my baby's health was worth a sacrifice, but I wasn't willing to give up things in order to improve my own well-being. What did that say about my self-esteem, my self-worth?

In the end, the gestational diabetes all but went away. My blood sugar levels stabilized, meaning I no longer had to check them daily. Emma was a robust eight pounds when she was born, perfectly healthy and normal. Getting to hold her for the first time, and seeing for myself that she was okay, I felt like I dodged a major bullet. And I was ready to indulge. I told my dad I would do anything for a Mountain Dew, and he was happy to oblige, racing to the snack machine down the hall from my hospital room. Emma was only a couple hours old, and I drank that twenty-ounce soda in what seemed like three long sips. Nothing ever tasted so good.

When Emma was about six weeks old, I went in for a follow-up with my obstetrician, and she ran tests to see if the diabetes was definitely gone. When the results came back that it was, I was so relieved. I vowed I would never, ever have to deal with that again, and I really felt as though I was on my way. Having

Emma and manufacturing breast milk was having a big effect on me: I'd dropped about thirty pounds in a month. Amazingly, I still didn't feel the need to binge eat—I hadn't returned to my bad habits. I was finally starting to feel good about my weight-loss prospects. My doctor warned me that with a second pregnancy I would almost assuredly develop gestational diabetes, but I shrugged it off. I was going to get the weight off before any other pregnancies, so that wouldn't be a factor.

∞

I'm not quite sure where it went wrong. I should have just gone back to see the bariatric doctor and resumed the phentermine to lose the rest of the weight. But I'd decided not to go back to work full-time and took a huge pay cut. I didn't think I could afford the medication and the doctor visits. Not to mention that the doctor's office was near my work, more than an hour away from my house. I couldn't make that commute with a newborn. Plus, I'd really convinced myself that I was now ready to do it on my own. Hadn't I stepped up to the plate with the diabetic diet? Somehow I'd found the willpower to do what I needed to do . . . I just needed to find that motivation again.

But find it, I could not. I wanted to start exercising again, but as with any newborn, Emma's sleeping was so unpredictable that I found myself too tired most of the time to do much of anything. I was stressed, trying to work from home and still make a difference at my job and trying to get the whole mothering thing down in a way that was beneficial to both my child and me. How did I usually deal with stress? This time was no different—I turned to food, slowly allowing in all the temptations I'd gotten rid of while I was pregnant. When Emma wouldn't stop screaming, I'd put her in the car—the ride soothed her to sleep—and the next thing I knew, I was at the drive-thru window. In no time my soda habit kicked back in, and I was back to drinking several Mountain Dews or Cokes a day. Predictably, the weight slowly piled on again. Of course that was when the deal making started, which began the binge-eating-and-regret cycle. I was right back to where I had been, and this time I was harder on myself than ever before. How could I not have learned my lesson after all this time, after all I'd been through? It now occurred to me that the implications were far more serious: I had a child to consider, and my health was very much an issue. This was no longer about wanting to wear jeans again or being an on-air reporter. This was about being around to see Emma grow up.

I could always count on some illogical thinking to come into play, and this time it did, too. Michael and I knew we wanted another child, just one sibling for Emma. In the back of my mind, I wanted to see how normal sibling relationships were supposed to work: bickering, yes; daily cruelty, no. I wasn't getting any younger, and I knew that I would need to go back to work full-time at some point. When Emma was almost a year old, we decided to get pregnant again.

It didn't happen the first time, this go-round.

It happened on the second try.

We announced it to our families at Emma's first birthday party. They were really surprised, and my mom, in particular, was worried. Two small children would be such a handful. Plus there were health concerns. I was heavier now than I was when I got pregnant with Emma. I was sure to develop gestational diabetes again. Would I be able to keep it at bay once more?

Again, illogical thinking on my part. *Of course I'd be okay!* I told myself. I did it the first time, didn't I? When it came to my baby's health, I was sure that I had what it took to do what I needed to do, period. I wasn't too worried at all.

From the get-go, this pregnancy was far different than with Emma. I had terrible morning sickness—I was nauseated all the time, and smells were my worst enemy. I could barely be around Michael as he ate his breakfast or changed Emma's messy diaper without running for the toilet. This went on for months, and it was debilitating. I was trying to take care of a toddler, I was working long hours from home, and I was trying to stay healthy, but it was too hard. The more I tried to avoid sugar, the more I craved it—and it seemed like the only thing that made me feel better, the only thing my body would tolerate. Nothing like a fizzy drink to calm down your tummy! I knew I was in trouble, but I didn't know how to stop.

I had to have the blood glucose test early this time, and of course I failed it miserably. I had gestational diabetes again, and I had to go back on the diabetic diet. I halfheartedly pulled out my old food diaries, once more employing the strategies that had worked so well for me with my first pregnancy. Only now it wasn't working. Foods that were okay for me to eat last time made my blood sugar soar this go-round. With my limited palate, I had very few choices, and I was always struggling to find something that was good for me to eat, that I liked, and that wouldn't make me sick. Every single day was a struggle, and I was miserable. The more desperate I became, the more I seemed to fail. I couldn't get a grip, couldn't pull it together. I was drinking tons of soda and eating carbs—all things that were bad for the baby and me. On the days I managed to do well and stick to the diet, my blood sugar numbers remained high. So I figured, *What is the point? Why "be good" if it isn't working?* I'd find myself drinking all the soda and eating all the bread I wanted, vowing I would do better the next day. My perverse binge-and-regret cycle had penetrated my pregnancy, and I didn't just feel sorry for myself—I was scared to death. My baby's health was on the line, and I felt powerless to do anything about it.

When I was about seven months pregnant, I got the news I had been dreading: I had to go on daily insulin shots. I swear, I wanted to run right out of that doctor's office and pretend I'd never heard those words. And if it was just my health at risk, I most certainly would have done so. But I knew that my baby's well-being was at stake. I had no choice: I had to do whatever it took to make sure he was healthy. I reluctantly attended a session with the diabetic nurse, learning how to measure the insulin into the syringe and how to give myself the shots in my thigh. Gathering my supplies, I wondered if I could get any lower than I was at that moment.

I had to check my blood sugar four times a day, and I had to give myself injections after each meal. With every shot I felt like such a failure, as if I'd done this to myself and to my child. I became really depressed, unable to believe that I'd actually let things reach this point. On my better days, I told myself that it would all be over soon; once the baby was born, I wouldn't have to do the shots anymore—I could start to get my life back. I never thought about the long-term health implications; I simply couldn't allow myself to go there.

I was increasingly worried about my baby's size. We've all read stories about big babies at birth, seen the television news stories about the fourteen-pound newborn. I started to have nightmares that I was in the hospital when a nurse hands me a five-year-old to take home. I so didn't want to be that mother, and with good reason: Big babies have a lot of health issues. Because my diabetes was not going away, I already knew Eli would have health concerns at birth. He'd have to go to the neonatal intensive care unit (NICU) so they could monitor his blood sugar, making sure it went down once he was separated from me. That was so hard to contemplate—that my child would need special care because of my inability to take care of myself. I wallowed in self-pity and fear.

Eli was due September 25, but I knew there was no way I'd make it that long. My doctor estimated he'd be about ten pounds, so she scheduled the C-section for the earliest possible date: September 14. I felt like I could live with ten pounds; both my father and Michael's father were that big at birth. And thank goodness I was having a boy—everyone likes a big, healthy boy, right?

I had such guilt over inflicting my poor health onto my son, and I just knew everyone else would judge me for it, too.

Labor Day weekend was especially uncomfortable for me. I was having sporadic pains, but because I'd never had contractions on my own with Emma (my water broke, but I had to be induced), I wasn't sure what exactly I was feeling. I called

Michael's aunt, an ob nurse. She said to take two Tylenol and take a nap. If I was able to sleep, then the pains weren't real contractions. I took the medicine and took a nap.

I slept for four hours.

When I woke up, I was groggy and sure that what I'd felt was some sort of fluke. I still felt kind of weird, like I didn't really want to sit down, but I just chalked it up to being big and pregnant. I had eaten dinner and started to settle in for the night when I started noticing that the weird little feelings were forming a definite pattern. I was having real contractions! But I was more than three weeks early . . . could this really be it? I called the on-call doctor, and he told me to meet him at the hospital.

I half expected to get to the hospital and be told I wasn't in labor, although the pain was becoming more intense. The nurses checked, and I heard them call the doctor to deliver the news: I was almost ready to push! Push?! I was supposed to have a C-section! I'd pushed with Emma for several hours but had to have surgery because she was stuck. I was sure this baby was bigger than she'd been—how would I get him out?! Panicked doesn't come close to describing how I was feeling.

The nurses calmly explained that the doctor was on his way and that they would do an emergency C-section. I immediately started to relax . . . and to get a little excited. I was so ready to meet my son, and so, so ready to not be pregnant anymore. And he was early! Maybe this meant he wouldn't be so big after all!

It was after midnight when everyone gathered in the OR. The on-call doctor wasn't one I knew very well, but I wasn't too concerned. He seemed like a nice enough fellow, so I really didn't mind—I was so uncomfortable, I just wanted the baby out, and I wanted him to be okay. As he was preparing me for surgery, the doctor looked at my previous incision. "Jennifer, I'm sorry, but because of the position of this baby, I'm not going to be able to cut you in the same place," he told me. At that moment I really couldn't have cared less, and I decided a little levity was needed. "Oh, that's okay. Not much chance of me ever wearing a bikini anyway!" I joked. This doctor didn't even crack a smile. I couldn't believe it! I could tell the female nurses were smiling behind their surgical masks. But Michael said this is also an important part of the man code: A man should never laugh about a woman's weight, even if she makes the joke. On second thought, I'm thinking perhaps that's the best policy.

As they all prepared for the surgery, I warned them that I thought the baby was pretty big. They laughed good-naturedly, saying they were sure they could handle it. The C-section was different than the last one I had had. The doctor was working harder—there was more pulling and tugging. Later one of the nurses commented they'd never seen this particular doctor break a sweat before, but this time he had. And we soon knew why.

Eli's first cry was healthy and robust. I didn't get to see him right away, but everyone assured me he was fine . . . and big. "I told ya so," I said, rather weakly. I couldn't see anything, so I was listening as hard as I could. At one point I turned to the nurse whose only job was to stand by my head and make sure I was okay and said, "I think I heard someone say twelve pounds."

"No, honey," she laughed. "That's not what they said."

"Twelve pounds, seven ounces!" a male voice gleefully announced from across the room.

The OR erupted in applause. Several people went over to see them working on my baby. I was in shock, and I think Michael was, too. More than twelve pounds? And he was three weeks early?

Soon they whisked by me with baby Eli in the glass bassinet. He was on his way to the NICU, as promised. I got to see him briefly, and he was a sight: big, red, and wrapped tightly like a burrito. He had a shocked expression on his face, one that I was sure mirrored my own. "Look at all of that hair!" the nurse exclaimed, pulling back his cap. Tufts of jet-black hair stood straight up. So that would explain all of that heartburn! Promising I'd see him soon, they took Eli away and I waited for them to finish closing me up.

In recovery, I didn't sleep like I had with Emma. I wanted to know how Eli was doing, I wanted to make sure he was okay. Because Eli was in the NICU, Michael couldn't go be with him, so he was as clueless as I was. Hours later, when they put me in a room, I found a nice surprise. The NICU nurses knew it would be a while before I could go down to the unit to see him, so they'd taken a picture of Eli and printed it out for me. There he was, with all kinds of tubes and wires in his mouth, his nose, and his arm. I wept, filled with worry and exhausted from the night's events. Michael assured me our son would be fine and I would see him soon.

Eli was born a little past 1:00 a.m., but it was almost noon before I got to see him. Michael wheeled me down to the NICU in a wheelchair—I was just starting to get feeling back from the epidural. I felt impatient as I went through the sanitizing routine before entering the NICU—I wanted to see my baby now! Michael wheeled me past rows of teeny, tiny babies in glass Isolettes—some no bigger than the palm of my hand. I was relieved my baby wasn't going to look like that, but I was also a little apprehensive about meeting him for the first time without the haze of a C-section and the bright lights of the operating room.

When I finally reached Eli, the dam burst. He was all alone in his little glass bassinet, no baby on either side of him. Truly, in this unit filled with underweight preemies, he was in a class by himself. I stared at him, memorizing all that I could about my new baby. He was wearing only a diaper, and his chest rose and fell so quickly with his little breaths. He was sleeping, but it was fitful, as if he were missing something—or someone. He'd been here for hours without me, and all I wanted to do was take him in my arms. Only, I couldn't. He was still hooked up to an IV, and I was scared to death I would yank something out or pull something loose. I touched his arm, my hand trembling. "I'm sorry," were the first words I spoke to my son.

Eli was in the NICU for three days, much longer than I'd anticipated. His blood sugar levels went down to normal pretty quickly, but then the doctors were concerned about his breathing. In trying to figure out that issue, they discovered a small hole in his heart—something they told me was pretty common and would likely repair itself, but a problem that would require more monitoring. In the midst of all of it, I somehow knew he would be okay. My usual MO would be to panic and jump to the worst-case scenario, but not this time. Something just told me that Eli would be fine.

I, however, was not fine. I blamed myself for his being there, for not being in my arms. He should have been in a regular hospital room with me, being passed around by cooing family members. Instead he had to be monitored round the clock, poked and prodded with every test under the sun. I couldn't forgive myself. When he was finally cleared to go home, when I could finally hold him and rock him and whisper lullabies in his ear, I still wasn't okay. My inability to control myself, to get a handle on my health, stared me in the face every time I looked in my son's eyes. And it almost destroyed me.

The hole in his heart did close. His blood sugar stabilized, and he lost weight. Every day, he proved to be a normal, healthy baby boy. I was so relieved, so thankful that he had been spared the consequences of my lack of discipline. I pledged to do whatever it took to keep him healthy, to keep him safe and happy. I became fiercely protective of him, vowing never to let him down again.

But I was letting myself down each and every day. I couldn't get my weight under control. No longer pregnant, I ate with a renewed vengeance, to the point of bingeing. I drank soda almost nonstop. On the surface it was my usual routine: I felt bad, and the only thing that made me feel better was to stuff myself with food, even if that "better" feeling only lasted a little while. But deep down I knew this time was different. It was as though I was trying to punish myself, make myself pay for all the damage I'd done. During my worst times of overeating before, I was able to pull myself together and complete at least a couple of days of better-than-normal eating, perhaps try a little exercise. But now, I couldn't get anything to work at all, not even for a day. I had never been this out of control, and I felt powerless to stop the path of destruction.

A couple of months after Eli was born, I got the news: My diabetes had not gone away. I was now a full-fledged type 2 diabetic. I wouldn't be able to put away the blood glucose monitor this time, couldn't disregard the diabetic diet. My blood sugars had improved somewhat since I'd had the baby, so I wouldn't have to have daily insulin shots. But I would have to go on medication—pills I would have to take for the rest of my life. And I would always have the stigma of diabetes.

I just couldn't believe I'd reached this point. I was still pretty young. I had two small children. And I was a diabetic. Forever. Suddenly I longed for the days when my weight was about looking better in my clothes or having a better sex life. Now my weight was causing irreparable damage to my body. And it was all my fault.

As is my nature, I reacted to the news with denial. Surely I could reverse this. All I had to do was lose the weight! Now that I'd had my last baby, I could focus on shedding pounds, on getting healthier. Once I got my weight under control, the diabetes, I was sure, would be a distant memory.

Surely this, finally, had to be my rock bottom. I'd had a twelve-pound baby, for God's sake. I'd been diagnosed with an incurable disease. Wasn't this finally the point at which I cried uncle? Wasn't I finally at the point to take charge and do something about it, for good?

Thus started my renewed attempt at getting diet drugs, and we now know how all that turned out. The whole time I visited new doctors and started new plans, I tried to ignore the diabetes problem into nonexistence. I didn't take my medicine, and I certainly didn't monitor my blood sugar. Doing so outside of pregnancy would have meant I was actually a diabetic, something I just couldn't face. In the back of my mind, I knew I was further damaging my health, but I forgave it because I felt sure I would soon get a handle on the situation—I was still deluded enough to think I would get on the right path. In essence, I let diabetes run amok in my body, unchecked.

I started to get chronic yeast infections—not just the "flesh-eating virus" ones under my stomach, but the more traditional variety. I'd never really had them before, and at first I was puzzled as to why they kept coming back. One Google search and I figured it out: Out-of-control diabetes leads to chronic yeast infections. I wasn't monitoring my blood sugar, but these infections let me know that the diabetes was as strong as ever. I couldn't get rid of them, and I certainly couldn't go see the doctor. I just sort of . . . lived with them, which of course, was insane, but so was my very way of thinking. It had been more than ten years since I'd started gaining weight, and I had yet to find a solution that lasted. What in the world made me think I would find one now, on my own?

Reality sometimes has a way of slapping you in the face, but for me, this time, it was a slow burn. I'd seen the commercials about people losing their eyesight because they refused to do anything about their type 2 diabetes. I'd read about a young mother dying from a heart attack, leaving her small children behind. I'd contemplate, more and more, how the deck was stacked against me, health-wise. My mother had had a heart attack when she was just forty-nine. My father had died of a stroke at fifty-seven. I'd seen three uncles die too early, two of heart attacks; two more uncles were being treated for heart disease. The odds were not good, and the more I allowed time to pass by, the more I let my diabetes wreak havoc on my life, the more in danger I was.

Looking at my children took my breath away. Emma was so beautiful, with big blue eyes that showed the world every emotion she felt at the exact moment she felt it. She was by no means an easy child, and she would need a mother's love to help her navigate her already overwrought emotions. Eli definitely had his father's temperament: easygoing, just happy to be here. But he loved me so fiercely, always seeking me out in the room, always wanting to be held and snuggled. Losing me would mean he would never be the same. Neither of them would ever get over the death of their mother. I didn't want that legacy for my kids. I owed it to them to find the answer, whatever it was. But how? How could I finally figure out what it would take to make it work, especially since I didn't know what *it* was? I felt like I was running out of time, as though I'd run out of answers a long, long time ago.

In October 2007 something happened that I still can't believe was real. Michael and I were in the den, watching TV. We'd already put the kids to bed, and I was doing my usual complaining about not having enough time to exercise and not making the best food choices. It was a conversation we'd had many, many times during our then thirteen-year marriage, and Michael's usual response was to listen, but not say much. Whenever I forced him to talk about my weight, he did so with great hesitation. He was so afraid of hurting my feelings or saying the wrong thing. Truly, I should have been grateful for this; I think everyone knows a husband who is anything but supportive when it comes to his wife's weight battle. Never in our marriage had Michael said one negative word to me about how much I weighed or how I looked, and I did appreciate how wonderful that was. But I must admit, sometimes I wondered, *What if he was a little harder on me, or just held me a little more accountable? Would I be better off?* At my worst, I blamed him when I couldn't get control of myself, thinking how he was letting me down by not being more of a coach. But when I was being rational, I knew what a gem of a husband I had, and how lucky I was.

So you can imagine how surprised I was on that fall night in 2007 when Michael broached the subject, all on his own.

"I think you should look into gastric bypass surgery."

I was sure I hadn't heard him correctly, but I saw the conflicted look on his face. It was one of great pain and reluctance, but there was also a sort-of quiet determination. He obviously didn't want to say this, but clearly he had been working up the nerve and had now decided there was no turning back. "You know Paul down at the sheriff's office? He's lost all his weight and he looks great. He said it was a little hard at first, but he's so happy he did it." Michael was talking so softly, I could barely hear him. At first he wasn't looking at me. His eyes were anywhere but on me—on his hands, on the TV. And then he turned to look me full in the face, his voice a bit firmer. "I need you. We need you. I think you owe it to us—and to yourself—to at least check it out."

There was so much I could have said at that moment. I could have told him I'd thought a lot about the surgery and had it in my mind if one day I needed it, if one day I determined I couldn't lose the weight on my own. I could have pointed out that there were a lot of negative things to say about the surgery, how everything wasn't as rosy as some people would like you to think. I could have listed a thousand different reasons why I thought I should have the surgery, and a million more why I didn't think I would.

But all I could do in that moment was look at my husband, who had so much love in his eyes it nearly broke my heart. All I could do was nod my head, simply, once. "Okay." Now it was my voice that was barely audible. "I'll look into it."

And that was all that needed to be said.

9

Life in the (Fat) Mommy Lane

I tell people how much I love to drive my minivan. I have friends who flat-out refuse to buy such a vehicle; doing so, to them, is officially cashing in every cool point they ever had. I thought I was one of those people. Before I had kids, I told anyone who would listen that I wouldn't be caught dead in the modern-day version of the "family truckster." I had a zippy little red Toyota Corolla that was excellent on gas and therefore perfect for my two-hour-a-day commute. It had leather seats and a sunroof, and even though I was way over 250 pounds, somehow I felt sleek and hip driving that little car. Mind you, getting out of the thing as a very large person was no easy task. I learned to park in such a way that I would not have an audience when I exited the vehicle—no one needed to witness that heave-ho process. And I avoided parking on inclines like the plague— they made it nearly impossible for me to break free from the front seat.

When I had my first baby, I dutifully put her car carrier in the middle of the backseat, because safety experts agree that is the best place for a baby. And because she was in an infant seat, it was easy enough to snap her into place and put the carrier on the base that always stayed anchored in the back. But what I didn't realize at the time was that eventually they outgrow the infant seat, usually at around six months or so. That's when you have to physically get in the back with them and strap them into a larger chair. And the babies are no longer quiet little snuggly newborns either; often moms have to wrangle, convince, cajole, even wrestle their children into the seat. It's a lot of work, not to mention what it takes to physically haul yourself in and out of the car. So when I was pregnant with Eli, I was relieved we had outgrown my zippy little Corolla and gladly gave in to the mounting pressure to get a certified mommy mobile. With a minivan there's no bending down, no heaving yourself in and out, all while maneuvering a squirmy child. It's easy peasy, if not very stylish or hip. Whatever. I was really in no position to fight for cool points.

As a very obese woman, I realized motherhood was going to be somewhat different for me. The extra weight I carried touched every aspect of my life, and I knew being a mother certainly wouldn't provide an exception to that rule. Heck, I even had doctors try to talk me out of getting pregnant while I was so heavy. And now that I've been pregnant twice while being grossly overweight, I'm not sure I disagree with their warnings. I wouldn't want to see anyone deprive herself of happiness, but I also believe that mothers have to put their children's needs before their own. I had to seriously question my ability to do that when I watched my newborn son in the NICU, in no small part due to my inability to put his health before my food addiction. Did I mean to cause my baby harm? No. But could I have avoided his being sick by waiting to get pregnant until my weight was under control? Undeniably, yes. There are so many things that can go wrong in a normal pregnancy, so maybe it is a good idea to avoid having a child while you're fat. Life as a large woman is certainly tough enough without adding carrying a baby to the mix. Not to mention actually giving birth and all that entails. It is, of course, possible to have a baby when you are obese, even morbidly obese. But trust me when I say it is not ideal, not by any stretch of the imagination.

Many doctors say the differences between a normal-size woman and an obese woman being pregnant start at conception. In other words, it's way more difficult for a heavy woman to conceive a child. The theory is once a woman reaches a certain weight, she stops ovulating. Having been told this by more than one doctor, I assumed it would take many months and a small miracle for me to conceive, but alas, that was not the case—I got pregnant right away, both times. But it didn't take long for the differences between me and my thin counterparts to crop up. It actually started with peeing on the stick.

We've all seen the commercials: Find out if you're pregnant five days sooner if you buy this certain pregnancy test. Anyone who knows me knows that patience is one of many virtues I sorely lack. So once Michael and I decided to try to get pregnant, I had to know immediately if our efforts were successful. So I figured those standard at-home tests were for chumps—I was going to get the test you could take five days before your missed period. I was going to find out as soon as possible!

So I bought the test. I peed on the stick. I waited. No second line; I wasn't pregnant. I was so disappointed, and a little part of me wondered if the doctors were right, if perhaps I was so fat that I'd stopped ovulating and it would be impossible for me to get pregnant. Sadly, I broke the news to Michael: We were not successful.

Only, more than a week later, my period still hadn't arrived. And I'm never late. And maybe my mind was just playing cruel tricks on me, but I could swear I was feeling some breast tenderness, one of the many early, telltale signs of pregnancy. I bought a standard at-home pregnancy test. I peed and waited. And it took forever, but finally, very, very faintly, a second line showed up. I thought . . . I was pretty sure . . . I was pregnant.

Before getting too excited, I called the doctor's office and spoke with the nurse. I explained how the early test was negative, my period was late, and the regular test looked faintly positive. "Sounds to me like you're pregnant," the nurse declared. I was ecstatic. My heart pounding, I asked her what she thought about the early test coming out negative. Did that mean that something was wrong? The nurse laughed, saying I was probably fine. "Are you very overweight, dear?" she asked. My smile quickly faded and I swallowed hard. "Um . . . yeah," I said, weakly. "Well, that's probably it, hon. When you're heavier, it's harder to detect the HCG hormone in your urine." I couldn't believe it. My being fat hadn't kept me from getting pregnant, but it had already inserted itself into my pregnancy experience—and had done so even before I knew for sure I was with child! *How else would my weight affect the next nine months?* I had to wonder.

In more ways than I could dream. I wasn't as heavy with my first pregnancy as I was with my second, but still I was about 260 when I became pregnant with Emma. So you can imagine there was no little pregnancy bump to speak of, no one coming up to me and gasping with glee at my burgeoning belly, asking me the due date of my blessed event. Indeed, me as a pregnant woman definitely fell into that category of "Don't ask." You men know what I'm talking about: If you don't know for sure a woman is pregnant, never, ever ask her if she is. That should just be man code, something they teach you along with how to aim straight when peeing or how you never complain about your wife's cooking in front of your mother. You just don't do it. Thankfully, I am most relieved to report, no one has ever asked me if I was pregnant when I wasn't; I have mercifully been spared that humiliation. But conversely, I missed out on all the happy speculation and surprise—I had to tell everyone, or always remind everyone, that I was indeed pregnant. Strangers really didn't know just by taking a look at me. And there were no cute maternity clothes to buy—no oversize tops to graduate to, no borrowing my husband's long-sleeved work shirts to wear to bed. My already limited wardrobe was now stretched to the max as my belly grew, and at the end I found myself shopping at the big and tall men's specialty shops. Nothing says "cute little pregnant girl" like a beefy T-shirt in 4X.

I was even bigger when I got pregnant with my son, not far from three hundred pounds. And I had the same problems with detecting the pregnancy in the beginning; I had to take several at-home tests before getting a faint positive result. But this time around, there were further issues. When I went in for that first vaginal ultrasound, the doctor couldn't see the baby. "You're sure the home test was positive?" he asked, and I nodded my head yes, my heart sinking. He called the lab, and the pee test they'd performed had been positive as well. Perplexed, he sent me to the large ultrasound room, where the technician was able to find the baby right away. The stress of the whole experience took years from my life, especially since Michael and I had announced to our whole family we were pregnant again just days before, at Emma's first birthday party. But I was relieved to call Michael and tell him everything was all right—because of my weight, the vaginal ultrasound had trouble detecting the pregnancy. And the same exact thing happened the next month: My regular doctor tried to do a vaginal ultrasound and couldn't see the baby. So once again I had to have an ultrasound done using the large machine, where everything was all right. I tried to take it in stride, but these little scares were stressful! By the third month my baby's heartbeat should have been detectable with a Doppler, but the nurse couldn't hear it. My doctor was called in, and she reassured me right away: Sometimes in early pregnancy, it was hard to hear the heartbeat, especially if the mom was heavy. I choked back tears as I went yet again for the big ultrasound machine, and yet again, everything was fine. I was barely four months pregnant, and I already had more ultrasound pictures than I'd had during my entire first pregnancy. If these early weeks were any indication, it was going to be a rough road.

I suppose there was a bit of a silver lining: I didn't gain much weight with either pregnancy. I wouldn't necessarily say it was a conscious effort on my part. In the beginning with Emma, I ate heartily, for once not feeling guilty about every morsel of food that went into my mouth. But then I was diagnosed with gestational diabetes, and the ballgame changed. I had to watch what I ate, and that affected my weight gain. I will say that my doctors never really scolded me about how heavy I was; it was as though they figured it was too late to worry about it so what was the point in berating the mother? I didn't feel pressured about my weight, and perhaps consequently, my weight gain was kept to a minimum. Score one for the big woman's side.

When it came time to have Emma, my water broke but I didn't have contractions. They admitted me to the hospital and started to administer pitocin. They outfitted me with a baby monitor, a belt that wrapped around my belly that measured my baby's heartbeat. What a thrilling sound that was! I'd spent most of my pregnancy a paranoid mess, always wondering if she was doing all right. Now I could lie there and listen to my baby's heartbeat all night—I found it so reassuring. Only, the belt kept coming unattached, and we had to call the nurse in there several times to hook it back up. Finally our nurse called her supervisor, a woman who was clearly having a bad night and seemed tired and frustrated. She started to show my nurse how to fix the problem, and I guess for a moment she forgot that I, the patient, was sitting right there. "Sometimes this happens with our big mommies," she muttered as she wrestled with the belt. My nurse looked mortified, and I guess the whole room, filled with my parents, brother, and other family members, just kind of stood there in shock. The nurse finally realized her faux pas, looked at me, and smiled nervously. "Oh, hon, I'm sorry." She truly looked upset, and I couldn't stand it. I laughed and patted her arm. "It's okay. You're just telling the truth!" I said, somehow anxious to make *her* feel better. She slunk out of the

room, and my mom looked like she was going to kill her. But
I shrugged it off. I guess I was too excited to meet my baby to
get worked up.

Despite pushing for a few hours, I was unable to get Emma
out—she was stuck in the birth canal. My doctor recommended
a C-section, and I was too tired to argue. Emma Taylor Joyner
was born, weighing in at eight pounds, three ounces. She was
beautiful, and I was relieved. I was anxious to try and nurse
her right away, and the nurses encouraged me to do so, even
though it would be a couple of days before my milk came in.
But try as I might, I just couldn't get Emma to latch on. I found
the whole process awkward and uncomfortable, and I'm sure
no small measure of that had to do with the fact that I'd had a
C-section and was incredibly sore, and it was hard for me to
move around in the hospital bed.

But being so overweight, I'm also sure, played a role; I just
couldn't get into any sort of position that worked. My breasts were
a swollen, misshapen mess, and my big protruding belly seemed
to get in the way of putting the baby in a position that accommo-
dated the nursing process. Bless Michael's cousin Jenna's heart—
she literally got in bed with me and tried to help me put the baby
where she could drink. It was horribly embarrassing, but I was
determined to try and provide my baby with the best nutritional
start possible. No matter what we tried, what position we went
for, we couldn't get it to work. I called in a lactation specialist, but
she wasn't expected until the next day, and the hospital nursery
asked if I minded if they gave Emma some formula from a syringe.
I wanted her to have my milk, but I couldn't get it to work and I
was worried about her nutrition. I reluctantly agreed.

The lactation specialist came the next day, and when we couldn't rouse Emma from sleeping enough to try nursing, she showed me how to pump. She also gave me some tips to try when Emma was more awake, but no luck there, either. They recommended someone else, and I was going to call—but admittedly, I gave up. I was too ashamed . . . I felt like I was too big and my swollen, disproportioned boobs were too weird. I decided, dejectedly, that breast-feeding wasn't for me. But I knew breast milk was best for Emma, so I pumped for three months. Yes, it was a huge inconvenience, and it made me sleep deprived beyond belief. I also missed out on the beautiful bonding experience I've heard so many mothers talk about. Eventually my body couldn't keep up the milk supply, and I had to let go of pumping. I did try, and I did give myself some credit for that. But to me, breast-feeding was just one more casualty of my being fat.

Pregnancy and birthing problems aside, I was eventually sent home with healthy babies on two separate occasions. And I am so grateful for that—we all know the myriad things that can go wrong, and I feel blessed to have faced relatively minor challenges in conceiving and birthing my children. But my weight was only beginning to color the experience of being a mother, in ways that I couldn't even imagine.

෧෧

There are the embarrassing, gotta-laugh-or-you'll-cry moments that tend to pop up everywhere in life, but more so when you are an overweight mom. Take the time Emma was a baby in the church nursery and I attempted to participate in a Bible study once a week. Regularly, I'd get called down to soothe my not-yet-walking baby—she was fussy and just didn't like being there without her mommy. Usually I'd rock her in the rocking chair while she calmed down, and eventually she'd scurry off my lap and crawl across the floor to play. When that happened, I tried to sneak out of the room without her seeing me leave and getting upset. One time I stood up so quickly, the snug rocking chair stuck to my ass. Meaning, I was too big for the chair, and when I stood up, the chair went along with me. It took some effort to wedge the arms of the chair off of my hips and put the chair back down. I wish I could say there were no witnesses to this spectacle, but you know that's not the case. Several of the nursery workers, along with a few moms, saw the horrible event. What did I do? The only thing I could do. I laughed—and they slowly laughed with me. I could have let it shame me into oblivion, but mercifully, I was able to find the humor in the situation. This, of course, was an exception for me.

There are, unfortunately, several pitfalls for an overweight mom to fall into along the path of motherhood. When Emma was just six months old, I enrolled her in an infant music class. Some may think it's a silly idea, but I thought it would be great to take my baby to a fun environment, expose her to some music and other babies, and possibly help introduce myself to other moms. Because I'd worked so much, at a job out of town, I hardly knew anyone in my city, let alone women with children. I thought this class would be a great way to have fun with Emma and make some friends. I just didn't get that it would be so physical. Emma was crawling at this point, so she was constantly scurrying out of my lap as we all sat in a circle on the floor. It hadn't been easy for me to get down there in the first place, and here I was, having to heave myself up to chase a baby, several times in a row, in a small room with no windows. By the end of the class, I was tired, sweaty, and winded. I was already self-conscious about my size; these conditions made it even more difficult to get comfortable enough to let my guard down and get to know these strangers.

Thankfully, I did eventually find some mommy friends to hang with, and boy did I need them. When Emma was barely walking, and I'd just found out I was pregnant with Eli, I was at a restaurant with an indoor play area for kids. There was a little toddler section to play in, along with one of those large indoor slides that bigger kids had to crawl up into and go through a maze of tunnels before sliding back down. The other moms let their babies climb the slide, so I shrugged my shoulders and let Emma do it, too. Only, Emma got stuck. And screamed. And I couldn't reach her—I was physically too big to get up there to get her. One of the other moms realized my dilemma and climbed up to retrieve my child. I was mortified. I soon learned to visit those places only when I had a very close friend with me or my husband—I couldn't risk having to admit to a perfect stranger that I was too fat to rescue my daughter.

I faced a similar situation with outdoor parks. I quickly learned to avoid play areas that did not have fences. Once Emma learned to walk, it wasn't long before she could run— and I was deathly afraid that I wouldn't be able to run her down. A very popular park near our house not only doesn't have fences, but it is near a very busy road. I couldn't risk

Emma getting away from me and my not being able to catch her. So we just didn't go.

Anytime we were invited to a playdate, I had to scope out the location and size up the possibility for disaster. Bounce houses? Forget it. How was I going to be able to climb in and get my child if he or she needed me? With my luck I would deflate the damn thing! You know how the mall has Santa trains at Christmas time? No way. I knew I wouldn't be able to fit in those little cars, and my children were too young to ride by themselves. So we only went when Daddy could go with us and I could feign the excuse of having to stay out and take pictures. And let's not even talk about the little chairs in the preschool classes. When Emma was two, her class hosted a mommy's day tea. All the moms were to sit at the little tables, on the preschool chairs, and have tea and cookies served to us by our kids. Only I couldn't trust that those little chairs could hold me, or that I'd be able to get up once I managed to actually sit down in them. So I stood up and drank my tea like a moron while everyone else sat, acting as though it was perfectly normal. No one said anything, thankfully.

There are literally hundreds of examples like that when it comes to being a fat mom. I remember seeing mothers sitting on the swings at the park with their babies in their lap, pumping their legs, going higher and higher to their kids' delight. Eli asked me to swing him, but I told him we had to hurry up and get home. I couldn't admit to my son that I was afraid the swing would break under my weight. I avoided paddleboats with Emma because life vests were mandatory, and I just knew there wouldn't be one to fit me. Instead of risking the humiliation of finding that out in front of a crowd of people, I feigned a headache and said we had to leave. At a birthday party, I told the other moms I got carsick, and asked if they would do a hayride with Emma. I watched on the sidelines as another mom held my daughter on her lap and I took pictures. I was too scared I'd cause the trailer to scrape the ground.

Probably the worst thing was water. It's been duly noted that I avoided wearing a bathing suit for years—I just couldn't bear "baring it all" in public. But what are you supposed to do when you have young children who can't swim? You can't just send them in the water and hope for the best. This may explain why Emma was two and a half before she ever saw the ocean, despite our living only an hour and a half away from the coast. The first time Emma and Eli stepped foot on the beach, I made sure I had reinforcements, taking along both Michael and my mom. They each grabbed a hand and took my babies into the water while I watched from the sidelines, fully clothed. The next year, Mom couldn't make it, and Michael and I took a day trip to the beach ourselves with the kids. I still couldn't bring myself to buy a bathing suit, so I watched as Michael tried to handle two toddlers in the surf by himself. He was more than a little annoyed with me, and I was so sad I was missing out on the fun. I knew something had to be done, but I couldn't imagine being in a swimsuit, weighing more than three hundred pounds. Friends would invite us to their pools, and I always made an excuse. I just couldn't put myself out there.

My biggest disappointment as a fat mom was pictures, or the lack thereof. When my children were born, I did the obligatory hospital photos with them, me looking dazed but happy alongside my pink newborns. And even when we first brought them home, there are shots of me outside holding them with the stork in our yard announcing their birth, giving them their first bath, or simply gazing into their tiny faces. But very soon after, I started to do my usual: avoiding the camera at all costs. I, as a fat woman, became the official picture taker. In other words, I avoided being in the shot by being the one behind the lens, which is really ridiculous when you think about it— my husband makes his living as a photographer, for Pete's sake! But I could not stand seeing photos of myself, hated the thought of leaving tangible proof behind that I was ever that big. Remember: In my mind, my situation was temporary; I was always on the verge of unlocking the mystery and finally getting the weight off.

Yes, I regretted not having pictures of me posing with Emma in her first Halloween costume, or a photo of Eli and me as he met the Easter Bunny for the first time. Pictures and videos of all my children's birthday parties will show my mother-in-law or my mom presenting the kids with their birthday cakes, waiting for the candles to be blown out. It's a job I should have done as their mother, but I was too embarrassed to get in front of the camera, so I stayed behind it. It made me sad, to be sure, but I figured, or at least hoped, that there would one day be plenty of pictures of me with my kids, once all of the weight was gone.

In my darker moments I beat myself up for once again letting down the ones I love. Of course my kids will notice I am not in any of the pictures. Will they wonder if I was even present for their big events? I put so much time and planning into birthday parties and Christmases. Will my children ever know how much effort I gave to make their lives picture-perfect, including leaving out photographic evidence of their big fat mother? I used my guilt to further torture myself, providing proof that in addition to having a husband I didn't deserve, I now added two wonderful children whom I had no right to have in my life.

In the moments I tried to feel better, I would remind myself that my kids were too young to realize what was going on. I didn't have to be embarrassed around them, because they didn't know what fat meant or that Mommy was morbidly obese. But we all know that kids are far more perceptive than we give them credit for—mine certainly have shown me that time and time again. One day, when Emma was barely two, I was on my way out the door to pick her up from preschool when I spilled Coke on the front of my shirt. I hastily changed and hurried off to her school. As soon as I walked into her class, she came up to me and said, "Mommy change her shirt?" She remembered that four hours before, I had worn a red shirt and now I was dressed in black. And she was two! *What else did she notice?* I wondered. *Could she see that her mommy was bigger than all the other mommies? Did that make any sort of impression on her?* I started to really contemplate what my being so overweight meant for my children.

I wanted to set a good example for Emma. I so didn't want her to struggle with her weight and her appearance like I had as a child—and I certainly would never want her to evolve into the mess that I found myself in as an adult. On the one hand, I was very strict with what she ate and the food choices that she was allowed, but what would happen when she was old enough to challenge me? How long before she realized I was setting standards for her that I didn't bother to keep for myself? And Eli—I know it sounds childish and stupid—but I wanted my son to be proud of his mother, to feel good about having me meet his friends. Were we that far from the your-mom-is-so-fat jokes among his peers? Would I see the day when he didn't want me to pick him up in front of the school, afraid of what others might think?

I knew being a fat mom would only grow tougher. Eventually I would have to put on a bathing suit, for heaven's sake. Michael wouldn't always be there to take the kids swimming for me—eventually I'd have to figure out how to get them to the beach and pool. And wearing a T-shirt over my bathing suit as a cover-up wasn't going to work, I learned. Years before I had kids, Michael and I went with my brother, his wife, and their young daughter to a water park. Normally I would never have agreed to such an outing, so afraid was I of having to wear a bathing suit in public. But we were on a beach trip with them for a week, and I really wanted to see my then-three-year-old niece enjoy her first trip on a water slide. Michael convinced me to go, and I agreed, thinking I wouldn't get in any kind of water, I would simply watch from the sidelines. Even though I'd managed to go the whole week without one, I did actually wear a bathing suit, just in case, but I put a T-shirt and capri pants over it, thinking I would never, ever take them off.

Well, I don't know what in the world happened to my senses, but by the end of the day, I was tired of looking at everyone else have the fun; I wanted to participate. Michael could hardly believe it, but I followed him and my brother up the big, winding staircase to the tall, swirling water slide. My sister-in-law and niece cheered me on, staying down at the wading pool to watch me slide down. I couldn't believe I was doing it, but I figured one time wouldn't hurt, and besides, I planned to still wear my T-shirt over my bathing suit. Plenty of people did that to avoid sunburn, right? For once, I decided to let go and have some fun.

We got to the top, and I watched my brother go down the slide, then Michael. When it was my turn, the young teenage boy manning the slide stopped me. "I'm sorry ma'am, you can't wear your shirt on the slide."

What? He said something about how my shirt could get caught and I could get stuck. I was mortified, but I didn't have time to stand there and debate what to do, there was a line of people waiting for their turn. I sure as heck wasn't going to draw even more attention to myself by trying to argue with the kid. I quickly took off my T-shirt and sat down at the top of the slide, putting my shirt across my body. I was thinking (hoping) it would provide me enough coverage.

Of course, you know what happened. The slide was twisty and curvy and wet and jumbled and I got thrown all around. Before I knew it, I hit the daylight and the wading pool in one big splash, legs all akimbo, my T-shirt crumpled in my hands, providing no coverage whatsoever. I'm splayed out like a Thanksgiving Day turkey, and the best part is, I have my whole family there waiting for me, taking it all in. Michael immediately stepped in to help me, while my brother turned and walked away as discreetly as he could. As gracefully as possible,

I stood up in the water and got the heck out of there as fast as I could, ringing out my T-shirt and putting it back on, sopping wet. Humiliating doesn't even come close to properly describing the situation. It would be years and years before I dared to don a bathing suit in public again.

Watching on the sidelines, fully clothed while my kids swam, or trying to cover up my body with a T-shirt, was not going to work as my kids got older. And it wasn't just water parks or Santa trains at the mall that I had to fear.

Before I had children, I learned that as a morbidly obese person, I had to avoid amusement parks at all costs. Growing up I had always loved visiting fairs and thrill rides, always game to try the latest and greatest roller coaster. As I started to gain weight, I suppose it didn't occur to me that not all of these attractions would be available to me. When I'd reached about 250 pounds, Michael and I visited Busch Gardens in Williamsburg, Virginia. They had a brand-new roller coaster at the time called the Alpengeist—it was one of those that ran on rails above your head and your feet dangled down. The lines were long and the day was hot, but Michael and I were excited to ride, so we settled in for the wait. As I looked around, I started reading all the signs that said how the Alpengeist wasn't for everyone and how you should avoid the ride if you were pregnant or had heart trouble. *Well duh,* I thought to myself. My own heart dropped to my knees, however, when I read the other signs. They said that "some larger passengers" might have difficulty fitting on the ride and that there was one row of seats reserved for "larger riders." I gulped. I felt silly, because it hadn't occurred to me that I might not fit on the ride. I hadn't had any trouble with the other coasters at the park, but this was a newer, fancier ride, and apparently it had restrictions. How would we know where the line for the larger seats was? Would I have to humiliate myself and ask? Plus, could I even bring myself to tell Michael I was worried about such a thing? I looked at him while he people-watched, oblivious to my worry. I made a comment about having a headache, trying to set the stage for a possible bailout.

As we inched closer, I strained to see where the larger seats were and which line we needed to go to in order to get them. I didn't see any signs, so I just started to look for "the larger people," and sure enough I noticed the beefier men tended to go to the row in the middle. As deftly as I could, I steered Michael toward that middle row, waiting for him to figure out what was going on. He was oblivious. As we stood and waited, I wondered what would happen if I was too big for the fat seats. Would I be asked to step off the ride? Surely that had happened before, but I couldn't even begin to imagine it happening to me. I would be so devastated, so embarrassed. My heart pounded and I felt nauseous. Michael finally commented on how quiet I was, but then went on to tease that it must be because I was scared of the ride. I played along, not wanting him to know the real reason for my fear. All I wanted to do was throw up and run away.

It was finally our turn. I got into the fat seat and held my breath while we waited for the harness to automatically come down. Mine did, and it fit me—just barely. I was safe. Michael didn't know any better. I'd managed another escape.

I knew a life with kids wouldn't provide many chances to avoid fat pitfalls. I felt I had to get the weight off—and fast—to avoid further embarrassment and humiliating my kids. Life in the (fat) mommy lane would not get any easier.

10

Last Straws

I'm a big believer in signs. Fate, destiny, religion—whatever you want to call it—I think it's real and true. Whenever I have a big question mark in my life, a crossroads I am trying to navigate, I pray to God for answers, and then I sit back and wait to see what happens. Surely something will point me to where I am supposed to go. Somehow, I will find the way.

When it came to the possibility of having gastric bypass surgery, however, I didn't want to see the signs. When I look back, fate was screaming the right thing at me, but I refused to hear the message. I'm not sure if it was stubbornness or fear or a little bit of both, but I just didn't want to accept that surgery was the route I needed to take in order to save my life. I ignored the signs for a long, long time—almost until I couldn't deny them anymore. Everything I tried to lose weight failed miserably, and at the end of 2007, I was very near crisis mode.

I was seeing a nurse practitioner about my diabetes. Actually I'd been seeing her for a couple of years, ever since my son was born and I was diagnosed with type 2 diabetes. She first put me on a few different oral medications and advised me to keep track of my blood sugar numbers. I only took the meds half the time, and I couldn't bring myself to perform regular finger-stick tests. I suppose you could call it denial, although I was quite aware of what was happening to me, both physically and mentally. I just couldn't accept that at thirty-three years old, I was a diabetic for the rest of my life—that my daily existence would involve checking my blood sugar, taking medicine, and saying good-bye to certain foods forever.

I kept thinking that there had to be a different way, a better outcome for me. I felt if I could just lose the weight, if I could only get a hold of my morbid obesity, then the diabetes would take care of itself, would disappear forever. Even though the nurse practitioner told me that now I was likely too far gone for that to happen, I simply chose not to believe her. I went in every month to talk about my "progress," giving excuses for why I hadn't brought in my blood sugar numbers. No worries, she told me, she would just perform blood tests to see how I was doing. And the news wasn't good, not at all. The various oral medications she'd put me on were not working, my blood sugar was way too high. Of course I wasn't helping things out with what I was eating and drinking—I was up to more than a two-liter of soda a day, plus all the high-carb, sugary foods on which I'd always binged. Each month she set out a new plan of action, and every single month, it failed. I was getting much, much worse.

∽

Enter Sign One. In December of that year, I attended a seminar held by two local doctors who performed gastric bypass surgery. I'd promised Michael I would look into the procedure, and even though I still very much felt as though it was not the solution for me, I knew that I at least owed Michael the effort of finding out more. Truly, I believed I would go to the meeting and gather enough evidence that this was not something that would work for me, and I would be able to take that proof to Michael, getting rid of the idea once and for all. To me, the thought of having the surgery was out of the question. And sitting in the lobby of the health center, looking at all the others waiting for the seminar to start, my beliefs were reinforced, at least in my mind. There were easily a hundred people there, and for once, I was not the largest one in the room! Sad to say, but that was a habit I'd picked up in recent years: scanning whatever public place I was in to see if I outweighed everyone else. Increasingly I found that I was indeed the largest person, and I would use that realization to further beat myself up. But leave it to a gastric bypass seminar to show me that there were, in fact, people worse off than I was. Heck, one person was even brought in on a rolling hospital bed! I couldn't help but eavesdrop as one of the coordinators explained to the man's loved ones that you have to be relatively well, physically, in order to undergo gastric bypass surgery, and perhaps now was not the best time for that person to be there. Yikes!

I was pretty nonchalant as I waited for the seminar to start, leafing through the literature, only half interested, really. I wanted to hurry up and get it over with so I could put the whole idea behind me. One of the doctors took the podium and gave a brief, generic welcome. And then he threw out a statistic that stopped me cold in my lined-with-denial tracks.

Ninety-five percent of those with type 2 diabetes who have gastric bypass surgery are cured.

I gulped. He had my attention.

The doctor continued with more impressive information about how a gastric bypass can improve one's life, and it was all well and good, but nothing spoke to me like that first bit of information. Cured! No finger sticks, no glucose monitors, no medication. I was now thirty-five, and I could be free of diabetes, seemingly for the rest of my life. I could hardly breathe, I was so excited by the possibility.

I opened my ears, and my heart, and really listened to the doctor, really read the charts on the PowerPoint monitor. It was mostly stuff I already knew, having read a lot about the surgery over the years. When he came to the part about the patient's responsibilities after the surgery, I perked up once again. If I were going to even entertain the idea of having this procedure—and I still wasn't sure I was—I definitely needed to know in what ways it could go wrong, what would cause it to be unsuccessful. I'd started to hear about people having the surgery, losing their weight, and then years later starting to gain the weight back. This was unfathomable to me. Why go through all of that—the risks of surgery, the expense—if only for it not to work? To me, it made no sense.

And then came the second stat that would stop me cold: The number one reason gastric bypass patients regain their weight is because they don't give up carbonated drinks.

That piece of news was every bit as breathtaking for me as the diabetic cure. No more soft drinks? Ever? Talk about unfathomable. There was no way I could envision my life without Mountain Dew. That sounds like a ridiculous statement, I know, but please understand: I didn't drink coffee. Soft drinks were how I got my get-up-and-go in the morning, how I relaxed in the evening, and what I used to drink in all the hours in between. I didn't drink alcohol, I rarely enjoyed fruit juice—it was all soda, all the time. I knew it had a lot to do with my weight problems, and it certainly had everything to do with my inability to get my diabetes under control. But I just figured one day, when I was finally able to get a handle on my weight, I would switch to, and grow to love, diet soda. I knew plenty of people who said once they made the change, and really stuck with it, they hardly noticed the difference. I just always figured that would be my story, too. But no, the doctor said carbonation of any kind stretches the stomach and a small stomach pouch is what allows gastric patients to consume less food. Years of drinking sodas could stretch it back to where it was before, a fate that I couldn't imagine living after possibly going through with the surgery.

I almost got up and walked out right then. Remember: To me, there was no way I could go through with having the surgery with any sort of thought that I would fail. And I couldn't imagine my life without soft drinks, period. As excited as I was about the news for diabetics, I really thought the no-soda rule sealed the deal for me as far as not having the surgery.

I stayed for the rest of the meeting, and at the conclusion I signed my name and phone number on the sheet for a possible appointment. But as I left the seminar, I felt resigned to the fact that this surgery was not for me, just as I had thought when I arrived. I had the evidence I needed to show Michael that it just wouldn't work. But I wasn't nearly as happy as I thought I would be. I left the health center and hit the first fast-food restaurant I could find. I ate the double cheeseburger, fries, and onion rings as quickly as I could. I didn't care if I smelled like fried food when I got home. Who was I trying to kid anyway? I was now hopeless and sad, convinced that the one ace I had in my back pocket, gastric bypass surgery, was now gone to me forever. Sure, I'd been looking for any sort of sign not to have the surgery, but I always kept the idea as a last resort. Now I was convinced my last straw was spent.

That night, as I once again stuffed food down my throat, barely tasting it, I didn't care what happened to me. And that was happening more and more in my everyday life. As another Christmas approached, I did my usual obsessing about trying to look my best for family gatherings and wondering what I would wear. Usually I would hatch some grand scheme of only eating ice pops and lettuce leaves for twenty-six days in a desperate effort to lose weight fast. Certainly not the healthiest thing in the world, but at least it was an effort, at least I still had some sort of hope of getting over this overwhelming problem. But this year was different. This time I didn't even bother. I ate whatever I wanted, whenever I wanted it. Sure, for some meals I would try to abstain, try to make better choices. But I couldn't manage even a couple hours of doing the right thing, I was so far gone. I was bigger than I had ever been in my life, although I didn't really know how big that was. I had long ago stopped weighing myself at home, once I found that I had maxed out the scale that we had in our bathroom. Yes, I was too big for a normal bathroom scale. When I stopped to really consider that fact, I was terribly depressed and embarrassed, so I didn't allow myself to think of it that often. When I went to see my diabetic nurse every month, she did in fact weigh me. But I explained that I didn't want to know how much I weighed, and she simply recorded it without saying the number aloud. My belly was too big for me to look down and see the numbers on the scale.

○○○

The news from the nurse practitioner that January was not good: She wanted to put me on daily insulin shots. My numbers were not improving (shockingly), and she feared for my health if we didn't do something to stop the blood sugar free fall right away. She tried to make me feel better about the situation by suggesting it may be temporary: Perhaps I could do the shots for just a few months to get my numbers back in line and then slowly wean off to oral medication. With good maintenance and a healthy diet, perhaps I wouldn't be on the shots for the rest of my life.

To say I was devastated is a huge understatement. When I was pregnant with Eli, I'd had to give myself shots twice a day. I found it demoralizing and depressing. Still, I did then what I had to do because my baby's health was at stake; that was not the case this time. It was just me my nurse was worried about, and I clearly couldn't be bothered enough to worry about myself. I recoiled immediately at the thought of going back on insulin; there was no way I could agree to that. My nurse, a warm, kind woman whom I'd gotten to know quite well, was quiet but adamant. Something had to be done, and this, she felt, was the only way. I left her office with instructions to come in for another blood test in a couple of weeks.

I pulled out of the parking lot and headed straight for McDonald's. The kids were having a playdate for the next few hours, so I did what I always did when I had some time and the house to myself: I got two double cheeseburger combos with two large Cokes. I ate one combo on the way home, and as soon as I'd let myself in the door of my house, I ate the other sandwich and fries. I then set the oven to preheat, already knowing the temperature needed to cook the frozen pepperoni and sausage pizza I would devour in one sitting. While it cooked, I checked the freezer, confirming what I already knew: There was ice cream left over from the night before. I'd top off my afternoon binge with chocolate chocolate chip.

As I threw the now-empty ice-cream box in the trash, the tears started, as if on cue. I was so, so scared. I couldn't allow myself to go on insulin, even if it was just temporary. And I didn't believe for a second that it was a short-term solution; that would mean that I would be able to get my diet in line and eat the proper foods. I hadn't been able to do that yet, had I? How would I manage to eat well when faced with the humiliating task of injecting myself twice, possibly three times, a day in order to stave off disease, to stay alive? Sometimes I thought, *I'd rather be dead.*

Enter Sign Two. As I stood there in the kitchen, belly full and heartsick, the phone rang. It was the gastric bypass doctor's office—they'd had a cancellation. Would I like to come in the next day? I wiped my tears and got out my pen, writing down the time. Yes, yes I would.

I'd come home from the seminar and told Michael about the soda requirement. I'd told him that I didn't think that it was realistic for me to give up soft drinks, and I really thought that was true. But he'd suggested that I should at least go see the doctor and see what he had to say one-on-one. I agreed, and then I promptly put it out of my mind. The holidays came and went, I was fatter than ever, and now my nurse was threatening me with daily insulin shots. I'd never felt so desperate. I still wasn't sure gastric bypass was for me, but I was ready to go and hear what the surgeon had to say.

I went to that first appointment still very much in let's-wait-and-see mode. But when I got there, I realized that my accepting the appointment made everyone at the doctor's office think I definitely wanted the surgery. At no time did the nurse ask if I'd thought things over or if I had any questions or concerns. She simply went about telling me all the things their office would be doing to get me prepared for the procedure, and all the steps I would have to take to make it happen. I know I could have resolved this by simply setting them straight, but I didn't, and I really don't know why. I knew there were lots of steps to complete before actually having a gastric bypass, so I guess I figured there was plenty of time to apply the brakes. After the nurse got my vital stats and gathered my insurance information, she remarked that I could have my surgery in a matter of weeks.

I was floored. All of a sudden this was a lot more real. Yes, I was still devastated from the visit to my diabetic nurse the day before, and I felt more desperate than ever to find a solution to this problem that wouldn't seem to go away, no matter how hard I wished it to. But a gastric bypass in a few weeks? The very thought took my breath away.

The nurse described all the testing I would have to undergo before the procedure: psychological evaluation, pulmonary testing, a possible ultrasound on my legs to look for blood clots. And of course, I still had to get approval from my insurance company. She told me she'd make all the appointments for me and call me with the dates, and she asked me to go to my regular physician and gather documented proof that I'd been morbidly obese for five years in a row. Sadly, I wasn't worried about meeting that requirement. But the other stuff just kind of left me speechless. The surgeon saw me briefly, and he seemed like a nice enough guy. I shared with him that I was worried about giving up soft drinks, and he reinforced what he'd said at the seminar: It was, indeed, a deal breaker. He wished me well and told me his office would be in touch in a few days with the answer from the insurance company.

I left his office more confused than ever. They acted as though it was a done deal, I was having the surgery. And I, stupidly, went along with it, for reasons that still weren't clear. Maybe I was still freaked out about the whole diabetes thing. Perhaps I was attracted to a solution that seemed so . . . permanent. At this stage of the fight, I was so weary, so tired of battling the same demons over and over again. But inside I kept reminding myself why I couldn't go through with it: *Having the surgery feels like the easy way out.* Although after getting more involved with the actual process, it was starting to occur to me that there was nothing easy about it. Still, I wanted to solve this problem on my own. To me the triumph was greater if it was at my own hand, not at a surgeon's. *If I have the surgery, the victory won't be mine,* I told myself. *Or would it?* Back and forth—that's how I went for days.

In the moments I was really scared, I looked for signs to turn me around, to show that this wasn't the way. I convinced myself that the insurance wouldn't go through, or if it did, that my out-of-pocket expenses would be too great. Since I'd decided to stay home with the kids and only work part-time, our money was pretty tight, and I really didn't think I'd be able to cover the bill for the surgery. Again, I was a believer in signs, and I kept waiting for the signs to tell me that having a gastric bypass was not the way to go.

Enter Sign Three: The nurse called a couple of days later to tell me that my insurance company had signed off; I would only be responsible for 20 percent of the costs. Normally this would be good news, but I was worried about that 20 percent. I called the hospital to get an estimate of the total charges and was devastated to learn that my share could still be as much as five thousand dollars. There was no way we'd be able to swing that, or at least that's what I told myself. I vacillated between being disappointed and relieved, it all depended on what the day's events were and where my mood lay. But in talking it over with my mom, she pointed out that my insurance probably provided an out-of-pocket maximum that was much lower than five thousand dollars. She urged me to look into it, and I did, although somewhat reluctantly. I thought I'd found the sign that told me what I was supposed to do, and here was another window of opportunity. And of course, Mom was right: My out-of-pocket maximum was well below five thousand dollars. The bill would come due right around the time Michael and I would receive our sizable tax refund. We could make the payment with no problem

I did have some pause when I received a letter from my insurance company. They reiterated their decision to approve my surgery, but they also wanted to make something clear: Excess skin removal was in no way covered by my insurance, so I better not expect it. Okay, the letter didn't exactly use those words, but the message was very transparent: If you have this surgery, don't call us when you lose all your weight and have a ton of skin left laying around. We won't help you.

I'd never really thought of this possibility. Sure, I'd seen documentaries where gastric patients, or even people who hadn't had weight-loss surgery but who had lost a ton of weight, were left with folds of unsightly excess skin. Many folks paid tens of thousands of dollars and endured painful procedures to rid themselves of this eyesore. Was that something else I would have to face? Would I go through all that surgery, recovery, and weight loss, only to trade in one bad problem for another? If so, I certainly wouldn't be able to afford to do anything about it; we were cash-strapped to be sure. And now my insurance company was letting me know there'd be no help on their end.

I tried to use this as a sign against having the surgery. To be honest, I was looking for reasons, desperate to find a way out of taking what I still considered to be a drastic step. How could I have this surgery, knowing it would leave behind such a horrible problem? I wanted to lose weight and feel good about how I looked, not be even more grossed out by what I saw in the mirror. I started to think that if I found a way to lose the weight on my own, through diet and exercise, then the chances of having hanging skin would be greatly reduced. To me, that was further argument against having the surgery. I started to work in this information with Michael, trying to set the stage for a possible withdrawal on my part. He didn't say anything. I think he thought he had done all he could, and he was just hoping and praying I would do the right thing. Only, I wasn't sure what that "right thing" was.

Around this time, we went to my mom's for a weekend visit, and my brother, Jimmy, and his wife, Mandy, came over with my niece, Chloe. I'd always found it really easy to talk to Mandy about my weight struggles—she never seemed to tire of me complaining about not being able to do anything about my body. She really listened, offering hope and encouragement. She is also someone who isn't afraid to tell you what she thinks, even if it may be a little tough to hear. I've always known this about her, and I think that's why I sought her out as someone to talk things over with, particularly when it came to weight loss. She'd followed my saga for years, and I'd been giving her updates about the gastric bypass journey by phone. Now face-to-face, we talked endlessly about the pros and cons. She asked a lot of questions, and I shared with her all the reasons why I wanted to go through with it and all the ways in which I was starting to think the surgery wasn't for me. She listened and nodded as I told her about having to give up soda and about the excess skin. I told her I couldn't face the prospect of having yet another surgery and especially couldn't afford to pay for it all by myself. I wrapped up my argument by telling her that the more I'd thought about it, the more I decided I was just going to have to find a way to lose the weight on my own.

"But Jennifer, how long have you been trying to lose weight *on your own?*" Mandy asked. "Has it worked yet?"

My sister-in-law wasn't saying anything I hadn't said a thousand times to myself over the years. And yet, hearing her say these words, at this time, made me really stop and listen. She was right, of course. I'd been trying to lose weight for almost sixteen years. I'd had minor successes here and there, but for the most part, I had been spinning my wheels, letting the pounds pile high and my health deteriorate. How long could I afford to let this go on?

That conversation really swung things around. Every time I tried to talk myself out of having gastric bypass surgery, into letting myself try to lose weight through my own devices, the arguments rang hollow. I knew I was at possibly the biggest crossroads of my life, and the path I chose could very well determine how long I lived.

The next few weeks were filled with various appointments. I had to have a pulmonary test to check my lung capacity; I passed. I passed a psychological evaluation, which ironically enough, was with the same therapist I'd seen years before. She told me she thought this was a wonderful thing for me but wanted to make sure I didn't have unrealistic expectations. I assured her that I didn't think having gastric bypass surgery would magically solve all my problems. I didn't, however, share with her some of the lingering doubts I had, basically because I didn't really think she would have anything to add to the discussion. I'd already analyzed everything so fully, it really was just a matter of making up my mind. And more and more, I was leaning toward yes.

At home I broke yet another toilet seat. Split it, right in two. It gave way under my weight, and it had happened more times than I like to count. How many toilet seats had Michael broken? Come to think of it, I'd never heard of anyone else causing this to happen. And yet, here I was—again—having to tell my husband about it so he could install another one. The sad thing was I couldn't even bring myself to be embarrassed anymore. I was starting to feel numb to all of it: the fact that I couldn't bend over and tie my shoes, the sad realization that I was too heavy to climb the attic stairs to put away the Christmas decorations—all of it. I used to cry and bemoan all these humiliations, but I was now starting to get used to them, they'd happened so frequently. And that, perhaps, was the scariest thing of all—that this state of being was starting to somehow feel normal, that it didn't shock me into action, no matter how futile that action later turned out to be. At least I would be making an effort. But now I could no longer muster up the energy to even try.

In my dreams, I was never fat. Even if a dream was disturbing in other ways, I was always the slightly chubby teenager, never the morbidly obese woman. That, too, started to change. I'd wake up and realize that not only was I heavy in my dream, but that my weight wasn't central to the dream's plot, it was just a matter of fact. That took my breath away. It was like my subconscious was slowly giving in to the inevitable. I was screaming inside, begging to pierce through and hear my own objections. But I was walking through my life as though I was underwater, and I couldn't hear or feel anything.

It was terrifying.

In all the years I explored the possibility of taking some sort of antidepressant, I was always asked if I'd had any suicidal thoughts. The answer was always no, and it was the truth. It had never once occurred to me that I should end my life—I never consciously thought that I would be better off dead. But in these desperate days, I started to realize that what I was doing to myself wasn't that much different than suicide. I was taking actions that I knew would cause me harm, that would eventually make me die. And I wasn't stopping those actions. I knew all the steps to take to lose weight—for all the hocus-pocus tricks I'd read about and tried over the years, I knew it simply boiled down to eating less and exercising more. But I couldn't make myself do those things, no matter how hard I tried. On the contrary, I couldn't stop gorging myself on greasy, fatty food, couldn't prevent myself from drinking gallons of sugary sodas. At the beginning of 2008, it almost felt like I was trying to accelerate the process, as if I knew there was no way I could make it stop, so why not bring it on sooner? Was I, in fact, ready to die?

Some people define addiction as a condition in which a person can't stop doing something that causes him or her harm. Over the years, I longed to be defined as an addict, because then it would be okay for me to get help. Addicts have rehab, they have medication, they have experts to help pull them out of the messes in which they find themselves. But our society doesn't recognize food addiction as a real condition, does it? The magazines, the television shows—they are constantly telling us that if we really want to lose the weight, then we need to pull ourselves up by the bootstraps and do the work it takes to achieve that goal. Any weight loss achieved through diet drugs or through surgery is considered less-than. How many times had I seen the cover of *People* touting stories of folks who'd lost one hundred pounds or more *All on Their Own! No Surgery! No Drugs!* I spent sixteen years convinced that I had to find the way, that my weight loss would only count if I did it without anyone's help. And now, at the beginning of 2008 and at some 335 pounds, I was starting to realize that I might not make it. I couldn't do it on my own. I couldn't stop myself. I was an addict. I needed help.

I continued with the necessary steps to have the surgery. I met with the nutritionist, I had the ultrasound done on my legs, I completed all the pre-op paperwork. All that was left to do was set the date. And even that worked out beautifully: The doctor could perform the procedure on March 18. My mom would be able to stay with the kids while I was in the hospital and while Michael worked—and then Michael already had scheduled vacation time for the following week, when I would be recovering at home. The money worked out. I passed all the tests. Child care was arranged. All the signs were there.

It finally occurred to me that my choosing to have weight-loss surgery was doing it "on my own." I was making the only choice I had in order to improve my health, in order to be around to watch my children grow up. By having a gastric bypass, I wasn't giving up and my weight loss wouldn't be a less-than effort. I was finally choosing to do what was best for me, no matter what anyone else thought. And that made me feel incredibly free.

Making It Up

I can look back at my childhood and identify the exact moment I lost any hope of believing in myself. As adults we can reflect on things that happened to us as kids and realize that they shouldn't have mattered so much—that in the grand scheme of things, they weren't that important. But even now the memory of the events of that hot July day back in 1982 still stings. Living it as a ten-year-old scorched my self-esteem beyond recognition.

I'd gone swimming with my friend Shannon at the local Ramada Inn. When she called with the offer, I'd jumped at the chance; we didn't belong to a pool, and the chances to swim that hot and sticky summer were too few and far between. The motel along the interstate had an Olympic-size pool, and local residents could pay three dollars to swim all day. It hadn't taken much pleading on my part—I was bored and climbing the walls; I'm sure my mom was glad for me to have something to do.

As much as I would learn to avoid the pool at all costs as an adult, I absolutely loved to swim when I was a kid. I excitedly went to put on the brand-new OP bathing suit my mom had bought for me at the beginning of the summer—only, I couldn't get it on. It was too tight across my belly. I pushed and pulled and stretched—and one of the straps popped right off.

Panicked, I called for my mom. Shannon would be there any minute to pick me up, and I didn't have another suit.

Frowning, Mom thought for a second and then disappeared into her bedroom. She came back with one of her bathing suits. "I can't wear your suit!" I protested. But my mom told me to just try it, and she was right—it did fit. In fact it was a little snug. It didn't occur to me then how sad it was that I was a ten-year-old who could fit into my thirty-two-year-old mom's bathing suit. I also didn't realize that the suit wasn't entirely appropriate for a kid or very flattering for me in particular: It was black with white horizontal stripes and it was strapless. I had no boobs, and my skin was freckled and pasty white—I was quite the sight. But who cared? I was going swimming! I was young and inno-cent enough that my appearance didn't yet rule my every action. Sure, I knew I was chubby; my brothers reminded me every chance they got. But my being overweight wasn't always at the top of mind yet, and I suppose I hadn't yet formed an opinion about whether or not I was pretty or attractive.

That naïveté would be gone by the end of that day.

We arrived at the pool around 10:00 a.m. We swam all morning on a beautiful, cloudless day. For lunch we ate hot dogs and chips at the poolside canteen, watching a group of older kids goofing around in the shallow end. I couldn't stop staring at this one boy in particular. He was at least sixteen and had a mop of sandy blond curls. You could tell he was the leader of this group of about five or six teenagers, and the girls in particular hung on his every word. So did I. I soon forgot all about Shannon and openly stared at everything this blond god did. If he was in the shallow end, I was too. If he and his group moved to the deep side, then so did I. I didn't try to join the group or anything; I suppose I just gawked from the sidelines. It didn't occur to me to be shy or discreet or embarrassed; I just thought he was cute and liked looking at him. Shannon teased me about it, but she agreed—he was gorgeous. I heard one of the others call him Scott, and I whispered the name to myself over and over. He was really tan and a really good swimmer. He dove perfectly off of the diving board time after time. Almost everything he said drew laughter from his friends. He was the most perfect thing I had ever seen.

Before I knew it, it was late in the afternoon and Shannon's mom was going to be at the pool to pick us up at any minute. The thought of never seeing Scott again made me want to burst into tears. As he floated on a raft in the deep end, a girl on either side of him, I hung out at the ladder, treading water and stealing last glimpses in his direction. Shannon was already out of the pool and waiting for me, but I couldn't make myself leave—I was trying to memorize everything about his face: his blue-green eyes, his sparkling white teeth. I closed my eyes and listened to his laughter, hoping to commit it to memory. I was having trouble doing that, however, because the laughter of the two girls was starting to drown his out. Annoyed, I opened my eyes to see what the problem was, and I was shocked to find myself face-to-face with the god himself. He was off of his raft and approaching the ladder, and there I was, dog-paddling and slack-jawed, directly in his way. The two girls laughed even harder from behind him as he made his way over to me.

I gulped. My face was red hot. My heart was beating so fast, I was sure drivers out on I-85 could hear it. I was scared, but excited. Scott clearly was going to talk to me—and despite my nerves, I couldn't wait to hear his voice so close to my ears.

"You know what?" he asked, his piercing eyes looking deep into mine. I was glad I had the ladder to hang onto, because I was sure I would faint dead away from his beauty.

He didn't wait for my answer.

"You are ugly as hell."

The glint in his gorgeous eyes and the sparkle of his smile helped mask his disgusting words, if only for a second. It took me a moment to register what had just happened. The gales of laughter coming from behind Scott jolted me back into reality, and the object of my desire helped me along by giving me a shove out of the way as he climbed up the ladder and out of the pool. He went to towel off and left his friends there, laughing and pointing at me. I swallowed hard, trying to get rid of the burning sensation in the back of my throat. I felt like I'd been slapped across the face with enough force to knock me down. It was as though my legs carried fifty-pound weights, paralyzing me in that spot of the pool. I was in shock. Soon my tormentors seemed to tire of waiting for a response from me; they moved to the other end of the pool. Shannon called from the gate to tell me her mom was there. My friend had missed the whole horrible exchange, thank God.

I got out of the water and grabbed my towel as quickly as I could, wrapping it around my body. I was pretty sure Scott and his gang had moved on, but I wasn't taking any chances; I looked down at the ground as I hurriedly made my way to Shannon and through the gate. I had been so excited to be at that pool and so sad at the thought of never seeing the beautiful Scott ever again. Now I couldn't get out of there fast enough.

When I got home, I told my mom I was tired and went to my room. I was so relieved to be by myself, behind a locked door. I slowly took off the towel and walked over to the mirror hanging on the back of my closet door.

It was as though I saw myself for the first time. I was fat. I don't think I had ever stopped to really think about it before that moment—never took the time to contemplate my physical state of being. But looking in that mirror, it was undeniable: I was hideous. My stomach hung in rolls. My thighs rubbed together like two large slabs of beef. My flat chest was accentuated by beefy arms that seemed way too short for my big body. I was covered almost from head to toe—my face, my chest, my arms, my legs—in freckles, and they were vile. My skin looked like bright pink bologna. My long brown hair hung limp and lifeless, stringy and sad. As I stood in my room, looking in that mirror, I knew I couldn't blame my wonderful Scott for simply stating the truth. I was absolutely disgusting looking.

It was one thing to be told by my brothers that I was fat or ugly; it was something entirely different to be assaulted with those words from a complete stranger, one whom I'd decided within two seconds of seeing his face was the closest thing to God on this earth. The way I thought about myself was forever changed that day. It never once occurred to me that Scott was wrong. I never thought to tell myself to brush off his words. Instead I took them deeply to heart, and they helped shape many of my actions throughout the rest of my life. Whenever I liked a boy, I relived that scene in my head, talking myself out of pursuing it. When my friends tried to tell me I deserved more than the abusive relationship I found myself in for five years, I told myself I was lucky to have any guy even look at me. When I finally met the man of my dreams and he tried to show me affection, I tried to push him away, remembering Scott's words and convincing myself that I didn't deserve the attention. From where I sit now, I am saddened that I allowed that pool incident to play such a large role in my life, but it did. I figured Scott had no reason to want to hurt me, no past action for which he sought revenge. He simply told me the truth, and if it helped him score laughter points with his friends, then all the better. I was uglier than hell. I was sure of it.

In March 2008, I was weary. I had been fighting myself all my life—never smart enough, never good enough, and never, ever pretty. I liked to look at my past and pick out the bullies and blame them for the way I was. My dad didn't show me enough affection. My boyfriend cheated on me and made me feel worthless. A beautiful stranger cut me with words so deeply that I carried them around like fresh wounds, even decades later. But none of those people were really to blame for the hurt that made me so very tired. I was. I couldn't give myself a break, no matter how hard I tried. Something deep inside of me resisted happiness as forcefully as I pursued it—and no matter how much I fought, my inner demons always seemed to win.

As winter slowly ended and spring began to emerge, I knew I couldn't fight myself anymore. I either had to give in, to let my inner hatred take over completely, or I had to take steps to stop the war once and for all. I couldn't do the push-pull thing anymore; I didn't have the strength. I finally realized that if I didn't step in and put a stop to it, no matter what it took, I would lose my life. If it were just me I was fighting for, I probably would have let it all end there. But I had two beautiful reasons to stay on this earth, and my children's existence alone led me to take a step that I never thought I would.

I had gastric bypass surgery.

I had waited sixteen years for my a-ha moment to strike. It never came. So I made one up. The lady in the children's boutique told me I would lose weight when I was ready. In March 2008, I was finally ready.

Now, that doesn't mean I didn't make the most of my days, presurgery. I had resigned myself to the fact that I would have to give up soft drinks forever; there was no way I was going to go to all of this trouble and have the surgery fail. So I spent the weeks leading up to the procedure drinking all that I wanted. And eating? Forget about it—I went on a "good-bye tour" of all my favorite haunts. Of course I ate something from McDonald's every day. But I also had a meatball sub and declared it my last, and I polished off a plate of barbeque and hush puppies and bid the food farewell. At my pre-op appointment, I met a man about to have surgery who said he had done the exact same thing, visited all his favorite places for the last time. Of course the doctor anticipated this kind of behavior and warned that if I gained a lot of weight before my surgery, it could be canceled. In fact they wanted me to lose three to five pounds before March 18. I wasn't so sure that would happen, but I did try to keep things under control somewhat, especially considering my diabetes. It was still out of whack, and the surgeon said if my blood sugar was too high on the morning of the surgery, the whole thing could be called off. Same with blood pressure. My doctor had put me on medication weeks before because it was high as well. So there were a couple of things to consider going into the operation, but I figured it would all work out. The day before the gastric bypass, I would have to fast, drinking only liquids, and in the afternoon I would have to start drinking some vile concoction to clean out my system. With all I was used to consuming in a day's time, I figured a day's worth of fasting would take care of most of my presurgery sins.

Once I finally made the decision to have the gastric bypass, I was pretty darn giddy. I felt great relief, as though a weight had been lifted. I sailed through the pre-op preparations with a spring in my step, telling anyone and everyone what I was having done. I suppose some people have some shame about having weight-loss surgery, or they at least want to keep it private. I figured I certainly wasn't fooling anyone; all you had to do was take one look at me to know what my life's struggle was. I was actually eager for everyone to know that I was finally doing something about it, instead of sitting around waiting for a lightning strike that never came. I was excited.

One bump in that road of hope was a conversation I had with one of the nurses at a pre-op appointment. She mentioned that she had had the surgery five years earlier. I was amazed— she looked great, and you'd never know she'd once had a weight problem. I peppered her with questions, mostly about what she ate and how long it took for her to lose the weight.

Offhandedly I asked her about side effects, and she hesitated. I could tell something had happened to her, and I pressed her on it. She reluctantly filled me in: She had a really bad time. Her newly formed stomach pouch had developed a leak, and they'd had to go back in to repair it. The second surgery left her sick for months, and she lost all her hair. When she'd finally recovered from that, doctors discovered a lump in her breast. Surgery and months of chemotherapy followed. She was all better now, she reassured me, and she was so glad she'd gone through with the gastric bypass. But her story gave me pause; I'd never really stopped to think about the possibility of complications. I had had two C-sections and recovered with little to no problems. I just figured I was good at surgery, and this would be no different. My surgeon had me sit through a meeting with other patients in which he went over all the things that could go wrong, including gastric leaks, abscesses, stroke, even death. At the time, I barely paid attention, believing it had little to do with me. But the nurse's very real experience left me thinking about what I was about to get into, and I was a bit worried.

I talked it over with Michael, and he did his best to reassure me. There was a risk in almost everything, he pointed out, and there was certainly a risk in being more than three hundred pounds, with a family history of heart disease a mile long. He told me I would be okay, that he would be there every step of the way, and of course, I believed him. I prayed about my fears, and then I set them aside, determined to stick with the decision I had finally made for myself.

I had to be at the hospital at 5:30 a.m. on March18. Surprisingly, I slept soundly the night before, all my nerves seemed to vanish. I woke up and dressed quickly, putting on no makeup and wearing no jewelry. I looked in the mirror, my face full of freckles undisguised by foundation and powder staring back at me, and I thought about Scott and the pool. I wasn't ugly as hell—I truly believed that now. But I was about to start on a path to be a whole lot prettier, and that made me smile.

I had Michael take a picture of me before we left for the hospital. I'm standing in the kitchen, in all my 336-pound glory. The first day of the rest of my life.

I finally believed that all the signs were pointing me to surgery. But perhaps what happened when I checked in at the hospital should have clued me in to how things were going to go.

I suppose on any given day there are surgeries scheduled for scores of people at any hospital. I was the first to check in that Tuesday morning for surgery, but there were lots of people behind me—some old, a couple of kids, some men, some women. Lots of people having a variety of procedures performed. Michael was told to wait in the surgical waiting room for me to be prepped, and then right before I went in, he would get to see me. The nurses said it would only take about twenty minutes or so.

I was assigned cot number one in the surgical triage area. Everyone is given their own nurse, and as lucky patient number one, I was assigned to Nurse Bob. I can't know for certain, but I'm pretty sure this was Bob's first day on the job. Or close to it. Everything he said, everything he did, was wrong, starting with the gown he gave me to change into. Imagine my horror as the front desk nurse overlooking the triage area called Bob over to tell him that I needed the special gowns that were in the second warmer oven. Bob looked perplexed, and so did I, until I figured it out: I needed a larger gown. Nothing like one last fat humiliation for the road! I tried not to let it bother me as Bob closed the curtain around my cot so that I could change. He also instructed me to put on a set of support hose—think: really thick knee highs. Apparently these were used to prevent blood clots. I changed out of my clothes and into the gown with no problem. But the little cot did not provide enough support for my big body as I struggled to put on the stockings. I tried standing and holding on to the cot for support, but it was too flimsy—it moved under my weight. I finally had to climb up on the cot and struggle to reach over my huge belly to put on the hose. I tried to keep my grunting and groaning to a minimum, as there were no sound barriers; everyone else preparing for surgery was on the other side of the curtain. Bob had to ask me two or three times if I was okay, and I tried to keep my tone light in answer, not wanting everyone to know my plight. I finally got them on and wiped the sweat from my brow. I was breathing heavy from the struggle, and Bob asked if I was okay. I already wanted to kill Nurse Bob.

The mayhem continued. Bob could not get an IV started. He tried one arm. Then the other. Then the first arm again. He was about to make his fourth attempt when the head nurse suggested calling someone from the IV team. My happy-go-lucky attitude was slowly draining away. I was now anxious to get this surgery started, and I really wanted to see Michael. The IV team arrived, and they, too, had trouble. I never knew I had terrible veins; my C-sections had been problem free. A sign? I wasn't sure, but it was too late now to change my mind. As the

IV team discussed my situation, my surgeon checked in with me, saying my blood sugar was high, but that it was okay for the surgery. That relieved me somewhat. He also assured me that they would in fact get an IV started, and they did. Now all I had to do was pee for a pregnancy test. *What?!* It's true—they had to know before taking me into surgery that I was not pregnant. Only, I couldn't make myself pee. I don't know if I was dehydrated from not drinking soda the day before or just nervous, but I couldn't go to the bathroom. So the nurse decided to give me fluid through my IV to make me pee. More waiting.

I'd now been there a full hour, and I was sure Michael was worried. All the other patients who'd come in behind me had already left for their surgeries; I was the only one there. I asked Bob if my husband could come back now, and he said, "Oh, I forgot! Yeah, he could have been back here long ago." To say I wanted to strangle him would be an understatement; imagine how I felt when one of the other nurses came back, looked at the stockings on my legs, and said, "Why is she wearing these?" Bob looked confused, and I felt the heat start to rise to my face. "Her doctor stopped using these long ago. He uses the plastic braces that snap in place." *What?!* I'd struggled to get the stupid things on, and now Bob was closing the curtain so that I could take them off. Shoot. Me. Now.

When the curtain reopened, I saw my whole surgical team standing there, waiting for me. I also finally saw my husband, who was just a little confused about what was going on. You should have seen his face when I told him we were waiting on a pregnancy test! Finally, I took the test, the negative results were revealed, and I kissed my husband good-bye. As they wheeled my cot toward the operating room, and the sleepy drugs started to kick in, I felt such relief. It had been a crazy morning, and a pretty awful sixteen years. I was ready.

I woke up from surgery with unbelievable pain. My throat was severely dry, and my bottom hurt from lying on the hard bed for too long in one position. One of the nurses beside me was clearly training the other, and I had difficulty getting their attention, as my voice wouldn't work properly. Finally I squeaked out that I was thirsty and in pain; they said they couldn't give me anything yet and we were waiting for a room to come open. I was beyond miserable. My C-sections hadn't been like this; I wasn't put to sleep for those, and I had a spinal block that kept the pain away for hours. Plus, I had a pretty, pink newborn to look forward to. As I lay there, feeling hopeless and hurting, I wondered, not for the last time, what in the world I had done to myself.

In what seemed like an eternity, the nurse finally wheeled me out of recovery and toward my room, only to run into my mother and sister-in-law waiting in the hallway. I can just imagine what I looked like to them—in incredible pain, no makeup, postsurgery. What a mess! They smiled sweetly, and I suppose I mumbled a response. To be honest, it's all a blur—a pain-riddled memory.

I was in the hospital for three days, and things slowly improved. Everyone told me how important it was to walk after surgery, but I did not want to get out of bed. I don't know if it was a side effect of the anesthesia, or just a means of escape for me, but the less time conscious, the better. I did walk that first night after surgery, and it did make me feel a bit better. But that next day, I couldn't shake my bad feeling. I was wheeled down to radiology so that I could drink some liquid and they could watch it go into my stomach. This test was done to make sure there were no leaks in my new stomach pouch. I passed the test just fine, but the nausea I had to endure from all that movement left me not wanting to get out of bed for the rest of the day. I struggled to find something to make me feel better, and I realized that all of the ways I used to cope in the past were now off-limits. In the hospital after my C-sections, all I'd wanted was Mountain Dew. And my very clear memory of that post-baby time, especially when Eli was in the NICU and I was worried, was that the soda helped calm my nerves, helped settle me down. Only, I couldn't have a soft drink during this troubled time. Whenever I'd battled nausea before, something I dealt with regularly in my second pregnancy, eating crackers or bread had always helped me to feel better. But I couldn't do that now. It really dawned on me that I had no way to cope, nothing to use to help settle my nerves. And that realization was very unsettling.

Looking back, Michael says he knew something was wrong the day I was discharged. My surgical wounds were healing nicely, and all the tests showed I'd come through the surgery with flying colors. I was packed and dressed and all ready to leave my hospital room; only, I didn't want to go. I said I was sleepy, and I proceeded to doze off in my bed. The nurse eventually had to come wake me, saying once I was officially discharged, I had to leave, unless I wasn't feeling well—in which case they would have to call the doctor. I reluctantly got up and got into the wheelchair to leave the hospital. Who doesn't want to leave the hospital? At the time, I thought I was just tired, but soon I would have more evidence that all was not well.

When we got home, I was so happy to see the kids, but other than that, I was pretty down. Despite all my research about gastric bypasses, all the information I'd collected before-hand, I was ill-prepared for how I would feel afterward. And the best way to describe that feeling is *empty*. I hadn't eaten anything in almost a week. I was supposed to be drinking pro-tein shakes and water, but the nausea was debilitating and I couldn't keep anything down. There was nothing to throw up, so I spent most of my time dry heaving, afraid I would bust out of my staples. I was nowhere near hungry, but something weird happens to you when your mind knows your body isn't get-ting nourishment. I would sit and think about food all the time. I'd plan in my head what I would eat as soon as I was able to: meatballs, cheese, peanut butter. I was obsessed with thinking about food and felt very deprived that I couldn't tolerate any. I also had a very hard time getting comfortable; the staples made it difficult to lie flat, so I slept every night in the recliner in the den. That, along with not eating, just made me feel . . . sick. And when you feel sick, you wonder if you'll ever feel better. It wasn't a happy time.

Ironically my house was filled with food. Whenever a mom has surgery, the community steps up to the plate. My mom friends, women at my church, and neighbors all brought tons of food for my family. We're talking fried chicken, pasta, cas-seroles, plus tons of desserts. Just the smell made my stomach turn, but the thought was even worse: There was all that food and I couldn't enjoy a morsel of it. I felt like an outcast. Of course, logically, I knew this too would pass and I would find a new normal. But at that point it was hard to convince myself that I would ever feel normal again.

Ten days after the surgery, on a Friday, was the closest I got to getting back to my old self. My staples were out, and I had a good post-op appointment at the doctor's office. I told them I'd had a hard time drinking the protein shakes, or eating anything on the liquid diet list, so they prescribed something for nausea. I was hopeful it would work. I even went out in the car, on my own, to fill the prescription and to buy some greeting cards. As I shopped, I looked at the people around me and realized: I'm doing normal stuff. I'm bathed. I'm dressed. I'm running errands. I should be able to eat something soon, once I take the nausea medicine. Things are good. I'm getting better. That night, I was very tired from my afternoon out, but I went to bed for the first time in our bedroom, out of the den recliner. It took a little bit to get comfortable, but I was hopeful, for the first time since I'd had the surgery, that things were looking up.

Cut to the next morning. I knew it before my eyes even opened for the day: Something was very, very wrong. Every muscle in my body ached, and I wasn't even moving. Lying still in my bed, I slowly opened my eyes and sucked in air. I was in pain. Everything hurt. It was an allover body ache, and it was scary. Still, I tried to talk myself out of panicking. I knew I hadn't been drinking my protein shakes or taking my vitamins as I should. I just figured my body was reacting to the lack of nourishment it had endured for the past several days. Vowing to do better that day, I made my way out of bed and into the den, where Michael and the kids were already up.

I convinced Michael to take Emma to her soccer game, sure that I was fine enough to stay home alone with Eli, who was then two and a half. He told me to call him if there was any problem, and I assured him I would be all right. I put on a Thomas the Tank Engine DVD, and Eli was hooked. I went to take a shower, convinced it would make me feel better.

Once out of the shower, I could not warm up. I was shivering so violently that I dove under the covers on our bed and stayed there for twenty minutes, trying desperately to find warmth. Eli wandered in to find me and saw me shaking; he thought it was a funny game Mommy was playing. I sure wish I'd felt like laughing. I followed him back into the den and put on another movie, then I lay on the couch. I was still freezing, and I knew I must have a fever. But I couldn't remember for the life of me where I'd put the thermometer, and I was in no shape to go on a hunt. Fever after surgery—that can't be a good thing. *But it's been eleven days,* I told myself. *Surely this can't be related to the gastric bypass!* I lay there fighting with myself, all the while trying to reach Michael on his cell phone, but I kept getting his voice mail. Desperate, I called my mom, who tried to reassure me from two hundred miles away that I was fine. In what seemed like forever, Michael finally came home and found me on the couch. He took one look at me and knew something was wrong. He found the thermometer: 101.5. I tried to argue that was a low-grade fever, but Michael wasn't buying it. He made me place a call to the on-call doctor. As we waited for him to call back, I started throwing up, or dry heaving. It was not a pretty sight.

A doctor who did not do my surgery was on call that weekend. He asked me if I'd had a flu shot that year, and I told him no, hoping desperately that that was what was wrong with me. He wondered aloud if he should admit me to the hospital so that he could do a CT scan to see what was going on internally. The thought made me panic, and I started playing up the flu idea. I told him that I felt achy and feverish but that I wasn't having any abdominal pain, which was the truth. He told me I could have an abscess, and I was flabbergasted. "Eleven days after surgery?" I asked. He said it was rare, but possible. I refused to believe it—I just couldn't. I asked if we could wait it out a little longer, to see if I felt better the next day, and he agreed. I vowed to take Tylenol to get the fever down, and I promised to call him back with an update.

My mom drove the two hours to my house to check on me. She agreed with me, saying it was probably the flu. No way would a complication of the surgery be showing up this late. Someone should have asked us where we got our medical degrees!

Mom had to get back to her house—my grandmother, her mother, was visiting from Alabama. She tucked me in for a nap and told me I'd be better soon. My mom always makes me feel better when I am sick, and I just knew this time was going to turn out like always.

When I woke up, the fever was gone, and for a moment, I did think all was better. But then I noticed I had a severe pain in my left collarbone/shoulder area. Had I slept on it funny? I wasn't sure, but it was sore and it really, really hurt. In fact it hurt all night, and the fever came back. By the next morning, when I was still sick, I knew it wasn't the flu.

I called my doctor at his office first thing Monday morning and he didn't hesitate; he wanted me to meet him at the ER. I so didn't want to go back to the hospital, but I was at least relieved that I would get some answers. I was tired of wondering what was wrong with me—at least this way, we'd finally know.

I checked into the hospital at 9:30 a.m.; I had my own room by 10:00 a.m. The nurses I had were really nice, and I thought, *Okay, this isn't so bad.* Michael was with me—he'd taken the kids to preschool and his mom was coming to pick them up and be at home with them, so I didn't feel all alone. I was still sick, but I was starting to feel better about the situation.

It was a long day. They took blood, they ran tests, and at about 2:00 p.m., I had to start drinking the nasty concoction one has to ingest before a CT scan. Keep in mind I wasn't eating or drinking much of anything—I'd had my gastric bypass only twelve days before and I still hadn't learned how to keep anything down. A couple of sips of the lemon-flavored elixir and I knew I was going to throw up. I tried my best, but I told my doctor that I couldn't drink it, I was too sick. He told me it was okay, they would inject me with contrast at the CT scan and hopefully that would be enough.

I was finally wheeled down for the CT at 8:00 p.m. I was exhausted, sick, and worried. The blood tests had revealed nothing—no type of infection. What was going on? I was still running a fever, and that horrid pain in my shoulder was still there. I didn't want any pain medication because it made me nauseous, so I just lived with the hurt. I was miserable. When I went in for the scan, the nurse stuck a cup of the nasty juice under my nose, hoping to get me to drink it. I almost threw up right there on the spot! I explained to her, feebly, that I wasn't able to drink it and that the doctor had said that was okay. She then left me on the table for what seemed like forever. I felt so alone, and I started to cry softly. *Why was this happening to me? And what would the scan reveal? Did I have another surgery to endure?* The very thought made me cry harder; I couldn't bear it.

All of a sudden, the cot beneath me started to move. I was headed into the CT tunnel, only no one told me what to do or what to expect. A mechanical voice commanded, "Hold your breath." *Was he talking to me?* I looked all around, but I didn't see the nurse, or anyone for that matter. I held my breath as the cot moved back out again. "Breathe," the voice said, and I blew out. The cot moved again and I held my breath again, as told. In a couple of minutes, it was over.

I lay on the cot again for what seemed like forever. Finally I heard voices behind me, and looked up to see my surgeon talking to the nurse. I had no idea he would be there! I felt better instantly, and that only intensified when he told me there was no abscess. In fact he didn't see anything on the scan that indicated there was a problem. I wept again, only this time from relief. He said they would run further tests, but I likely just had the flu or some other bug. I could go home in the morning.

When a guy from the transport team came to wheel me back to my room, he saw me crying and asked if I was okay. "Yes! My scan was clear. I am so happy!" I told him. He laughed. "Of course you're okay, honey. God's got you."

His words enveloped me like a warm hug. I felt more hopeful than I had in a while.

I was discharged the next day. I was so hopeful, I didn't want to wait for the wheelchair to take me out of the hospital. Walking out on my own symbolized to me that I was on the road to recovery. And I did feel a little better when I got home. But the stubborn pain in my collarbone area soon came back and hurt worse than ever.

I had a follow-up appointment scheduled with my surgeon. As I sat in his waiting room, I had to keep my ice-cold water bottle on my collarbone—that was the only way I could get some relief. When I saw the doctor, I told him the fever was gone but that the awful pain was still there, throbbing. He didn't know right away what could be causing the pain, so he ordered more tests. He asked if I was eating and drinking and I lied, telling him yes. The truth was I still couldn't stomach the awful protein shakes, and I was only taking my vitamins half the time. I still battled crippling nausea, and I was worried that even when they were cut in half, the pills were too big for my tiny stomach pouch. He promised to call with the results of the tests, and he sent me on my way.

I only had a couple of hours before I had to pick up the kids from preschool, and I was worried. This would be my first time alone with my children since before the surgery, and I was in so much pain, I didn't know how I would manage. If only I could get some pain relief! I thought about the Percocet I had at home. Maybe if I could force myself to eat a little something, I could take the pain medicine without throwing up. And maybe the pain relief would be enough to get me through the afternoon with the kids until Michael got home. That's what I was reduced to—just trying to make it through the day.

And so it was that my first food after surgery was ... mashed potatoes. I stopped at Bojangles' and got some, sans gravy. Here it was, almost fifteen days since my gastric bypass, and this was the first real food I'd had. And I was so scared . . . of getting sick, of the food getting *stuck*. But at that point, I would have done anything to make that pain go away, even take pain medication I had managed to avoid after two C-sections. Enough was enough.

I was able to eat four to five bites of the potatoes. And I took two Percocet when I got home. In less than thirty minutes, I was soaring. My mind was mushy, and I felt removed from my body. It was a disconcerting feeling, especially when I was about to go drive in a car and pick up my kids. But I had to get away from that pain, whatever it took.

The next two days were a blur. I somehow went about my daily life, doing my job, which meant recording radio newscasts from my home computer, taking the kids to preschool, picking them up, making dinner. I was in pain, and the fever came back. I felt just as sick as I always had. The only time I got some relief was when I took the pain medicine. Not only did it alleviate some of the physical pain in my collarbone, it left me in such a fog, I was able not to feel . . . anything. It kept at bay some of the rising doubts in my mind: *Was the surgery a mistake? Would I ever feel better? Was this any way to live?* These questions were way too heavy for me; I just wanted to escape.

I was shutting out all my friends and family. I don't think I did it on purpose; I just didn't know what to say to them. They all wanted to know if I was feeling better, and I knew that if I told them no, I was feeling worse, the inevitable follow-up questions would be, "What's wrong?" and "What are you doing about it?" I didn't know what was wrong, and my doctor wasn't doing anything about it. I was starting to feel like I was crazy. All my mom friends knew I was having trouble, and offers of food for the family and help with child care were still pouring in. I ignored most of them, because I didn't know how to respond, what to think. At the preschool one day, one of the well-meaning moms asked if I wanted to speak to her friend, Lisa, who had just had the surgery a week before me and was doing great. Uh, no, I didn't want to speak to her—I cut the poor woman off and practically ran away. She meant well, but I didn't need to be reminded that I was a freak, someone who statistically speaking should be doing fine by now but who was beyond miserable.

That afternoon, I became aware of how incapable I was of being a caregiver for my children. I wasn't supposed to lift anything for a couple of weeks, and that meant not picking up the children. I got around this in various ways, including having Eli step up into a chair and climb over the crib railing when it was time for his nap. Probably not the safest thing in the world, but he was two and a half, and I stood right there while he did it, sure that I would be able to help if needed. While both kids were sleeping, I writhed around in agony, my collarbone pain hurting so much, I was near tears. It wasn't long before Eli woke up and wanted out of his crib. I couldn't let him climb out the same way he'd climbed in; even I knew that was too dangerous. The day before, I'd been able to lift him out, even though I wasn't supposed to and it hurt like hell. This day, however, I just couldn't do it. I could barely lift my arms, much less a thirty-pound toddler. So at first I ignored his cries, hoping he would fall back asleep. When he only got louder, I walked to his room, doubled over from the pain. Feebly I tried to soothe him with my words, but honestly, I thought I would die . . . and I was scared. I couldn't even care for my child! There I sat with him, for forty-five minutes, talking to him and playing with him through the slats of his crib. Michael eventually got home, and I tearfully told him how I wasn't able to lift our son out of his crib.

Finally I couldn't take it any longer. I called the doctor's office and told his nurse that my pain was worse than ever and the fever was back. I couldn't function in my daily life, and I needed help. She called back that evening, saying the surgeon wanted me to have another CT scan, this time as an outpatient. I went the next day and had a much better experience. I wasn't made to drink anything yucky, and the nurse gave me complete instructions on what to do. That afternoon the surgeon's nurse called me at home with the results: no abscess. Nothing wrong that they could see. I probably just had a bug and would feel better in a few days. "But what about the pain in my collarbone?" I asked weakly. The nurse wasn't sure, but she scheduled an appointment for me to see the doctor in a couple of days.

That night Michael was furious. He couldn't believe the doctor wasn't doing more and that I was still in so much pain. As I sat in the recliner, I thought I would faint from the pain in my shoulder area. Michael gave me more pain meds, and they helped. We reluctantly made plans to send the kids off—Emma would go to my mom's house and Eli would go to Michael's parents. It broke our hearts to do this—our children had never been away from both of us, not even for one night. Michael would go with me to the doctor, and he vowed not to leave until we found out something definitive.

We went to the surgeon's office and didn't have to wait long. As we waited for the doctor, I tearfully told the nurse that I wasn't any better and I desperately needed some help. As if on cue my doctor came in the room, and I swear he was whistling, as though he didn't have a care in the world. He stopped abruptly when he saw me start to cry even harder. I couldn't speak, so Michael told him I wasn't feeling any better and that my pain was in fact a lot worse. It was then that the doctor said he hadn't read the latest CT scan himself; he simply went by what the radiologist told him, that the scan was clear. He left the exam room to go pull up the report to get a look for himself.

He was back in less than five minutes, phone to his ear. "I'm calling the radiologist now. I see an abscess."

The news should have been devastating, but all I could feel was relief. So I wasn't crazy! I'd known that something wasn't right, and now there was proof to back me up. Even if it meant another stay in the hospital, and a painful procedure to endure, I was relieved to finally have some answers.

My relief was short-lived. I had to report back to the hospital the next morning for a CT-guided drain of the abscess. They would use the CT machine to find the infection, and then the radiologist would use a very long needle to get the liquid out. I would be awake the entire time, and they would not be able to give me a lot for the pain because I had to be awake and alert for the procedure.

Fabulous.

I was already in a lot of pain. But I was told not to eat or drink anything after midnight, so I went in, having had no pain medication. I was really hurting. The nurse who was going to be with me for the procedure was apparently having a bad day. She shuffled her feet slowly to complete her tasks, taking her sweet time. I was in agony. She then told me to lie down on the cot and to not move. This was unreal to me—since the pain in my collarbone had arrived, I'd been sleeping in the recliner again, unable to lie flat because of the pain. Now she wanted me to lie there and not move a muscle. Excruciating.

So I lay there while she did a bunch of stuff. And I lay there while she talked to some people. And I lay there while she disappeared for a while. With tears streaming down my face, I asked her, when she came back, what we were waiting for, and she said we were waiting for the radiologist to arrive. I asked her if I could get up until he got there, just to stretch and try to relieve some of the pain, but she said no—it was very important that I keep the same position. I really thought I would die, I hurt so much.

Another fifteen minutes or so went by. She then breezed in and told me that after the procedure I would be going to a stepdown unit to be monitored, and then I would be sent home. *What?* I told her that my doctor said I would be in the hospital for several days—that he wanted to make sure this time there were no more complications. Believe me, even though I now hated hospitals with a passion, I wholly supported that idea, after all I'd been through. But this nurse told me that my doctor wasn't in charge of the whole hospital and that there simply weren't enough beds for me to stay. I was going home, and that was that. I cried even more. She then told me that if I wanted to,

I could go call my doctor for confirmation. This time I couldn't hold back. "Oh! *Now* you'll let me get down? I've been writhing in pain for more than an hour, begging you to let me move, and you said no, I had to stay in the same position! *Now you're going to let me get down?*" I didn't know how to call my doctor—it wasn't like I carried his phone number with me. I just cried harder, scared and in pain, not knowing what to do. The nurse left me there.

I'd made up my mind to put a stop to the whole thing when the radiologist walked in the door. He looked at me and knew I was in pain and was very kind. He told me he was sorry that things were taking so long, that he'd been conferencing with my surgeon and wanted to make sure he had all he needed before the procedure. He promised it wouldn't be long before he was finished and I could have something for the pain.

It was the worst experience of my life. It hurt so much, and it made me nauseous. I lay on that table, begging for it to be over. The nurse who'd been so unkind to me held my hand and looked a bit remorseful. Finally the procedure was complete. The doctor would later tell my husband that they took out more than a liter of fluid.

The radiologist made sure I got pain medication as soon as the procedure was over. They brought Michael in, and I told him what the nurse said about my leaving the hospital. He was as mad as I was, and he went to find my doctor. As I lay on the cot, I started to shiver uncontrollably, and the previously unkind nurse went to get me more blankets. When my doctor came in, I was shaking so hard it was difficult to talk. But he assured me I had a room and that I wasn't going anywhere.

Had I felt any better, I would have smirked at the nurse when I was wheeled away.

The hope was that I would start to improve right away once the liquid had been drained. But my fever came back, and my oxygen levels were not great. Also, I was starting to have difficulty breathing—shortness of breath when I got up to go to the bathroom and some pain when I was asked to breathe deeply. The doctor ordered a chest X-ray, and a pulmonologist was called.

I also had trouble with my IV. That came as no surprise to me; in addition to my earlier problems, I was sure I was quite dehydrated at this point. This was now the weekend, and another doctor instead of my surgeon was on call. He told me they would have to put in a central line because my IV kept blowing out. Honestly, I felt so crummy at that point, I didn't really care. Michael stepped out of the room while the doctor tried to put in the line, but he was having trouble. It hurt so much, but I tried not to cry—I could feel this doctor's unease, and I didn't want to shake his confidence. He said he was taking a break and would be back in a minute to try the other side. The nurse said she was going to change my bedding, and she wanted me not to look down at my sheets. Michael, who came to be with me while the doctor was out, told me later that my bed had been full of blood.

The doctor was finally able to establish the central line, and I suppose that was one less thing I had to worry about. Of course, I had blood in my hair—and no prospects of a shower anytime soon—but I really didn't care. I was so demoralized at that point; it was difficult for me to get upset about anything.

The pulmonologist said my left lung was filled with fluid and that I had to do around-the-clock breathing treatments to get it under control. I couldn't be bothered. I lived to take the pain medicine every four hours. That pain medicine made me sleepy, and sleep helped me escape the situation. All I wanted was to not be conscious, not have to live this nightmare. Michael was by my side, trying to force me to do what the doctor said. I gave it a halfhearted try, but I really didn't care. Michael was starting to feel guilty. He was blaming himself for what was happening to me, wondering if he hadn't raised the idea of gastric bypass surgery, would we even be in this situation. I tried to reassure him, but honestly I was too sick. I couldn't do much of anything.

On Monday my doctor was back, and he told me I'd have to have a chest tube inserted. My lung was partially collapsed from all the fluid underneath. All I could think about was that it sounded like another painful procedure; if it was anything like the CT-guided drain of the abscess, then I didn't think I'd survive. The doctor said I did, in fact, have to be awake for the chest tube insertion. I just started bawling. I couldn't face it, couldn't take any more pain. My doctor assured Michael that I would be fine—and he was right. They gave me something that left me with no memory of the procedure. Michael said I came back, loopy and happy. I also had a tube coming out of my side, attached to a ten-pound box that would carry the drainage. It made getting out of bed very tricky, and painful. Over the next few days, I learned to time my visits to the bathroom around my pain medication. And I had to make sure the nurse also gave me nausea medicine with the pain meds, because I certainly wasn't eating. Every mealtime a tray of food was delivered to my room, and every time it sat, untouched. The doctor asked how I was eating, and I told him I was fine. I certainly wasn't hungry, and now, almost twenty days after the surgery, I was almost used to not eating. Michael kept gently reminding me that I would never get better if my body didn't have nourishment, but he didn't push too hard. He knew I felt like crap, and he still felt guilty. I just figured I'd eat eventually . . . or . . . not. I still didn't care.

At one point the kids came back. My mother-in-law snuck Eli into the hospital to see me, but I was wracked with pain and could barely enjoy the visit. Michael had to go back to work, and my mother-in-law took the kids to school, picked them up, and stayed with them at my house until Michael got home. I felt as though life was going on without me, and that just added fuel to my self-pity fire. It was hard to get better when I felt so miserable.

I'm pretty sure I was a difficult patient, and I couldn't have been that much fun to be around. But I must say, the way some of the nurses treated me was appalling. I'd heard this was the case with gastric bypass patients, and I have to admit, in my experience, it was true. For the most part I found them to be unsympathetic and sometimes downright rude. My chest tube was inserted on my left side, but I had to get out of bed on the right. When I had to go to the bathroom, I had to call a nurse in and have her hold both of my hands while I pulled myself up, slowly. I then had the nurse stay while I swung my legs around and lifted myself out of bed, negotiating the ten-pound box attached to the tube, plus all my surgical wounds. It was an ordeal. I had one nurse say to me, "I can't help you. I'm sorry, but I can't risk hurting myself." *What?* I wasn't asking her to lift me out of bed, for goodness' sake! Plus, could she have told me this before I was half hanging off the bed? I struggled to get up without her help, in incredible pain. It was a nightmare.

There were a couple of exceptions—mostly nursing assistants whose job it was to take my blood pressure, temperature, and so on. There was one in particular who always took the time to ask how I was doing, to see if she could get anything for me. One day, while I was asleep, she left me some shampoo that can be used without water. She knew it had been a week since I'd bathed, and I still had blood stuck in my hair from when they had to establish the central line for my IV. I later found out that this nursing assistant had gone to the drugstore on her own time to get me that shampoo. That meant a lot.

Finally, after eight days, it was time to go home. My lung had reinflated, and all the follow-up testing said the abscess had abated. I was scared to death of having the chest tube taken out, and my doctor's physician's assistant made no bones about it when she told me it was going to hurt. But she looked at my orders and discovered my doctor had authorized morphine. With my central line still in place, it was no time before the nurse had given me a morphine shot, on top of the pain meds I had just taken. The chest tube came out with little discomfort, and I was finally ready to go home.

I had mixed feelings. I missed my children so much; they'd never spent a night away from home, and Michael and I both felt bad that they'd had to go live with their grandparents for a week. Of course they had a blast, and that certainly made me feel better. I wanted to touch them and hug them and let them know that Mommy was home and going to be better. But was I? I was so weak, I not only had to wait for the wheelchair to take me out of the hospital, I had trouble getting into the car. My muscles had atrophied, and I had no strength whatsoever. And of course that wasn't helped by the fact that I still wasn't eating. When I was discharged, the physician's assistant gave me the go-ahead to slowly introduce soft solids into my diet. Little did she know I still wasn't past the liquid stage! No vitamins, no protein shakes, and very little water. I was a mess.

As we walked in the front door and my children ran over to me, I closed my eyes and took in their smell. "Mommy's home," I said to them, getting gentle hugs and kisses. *But will I ever feel the same?* I wondered.

12

Shipwrecked

I spend my thirty-sixth birthday in a ratty old recliner in our den, wearing the same pajamas from two days before and not bothering to brush my hair or wash my face. Beside me is my son's Lego table, which has become my medical nightstand: It holds all my pills, a barely touched bottle of water, and a fan to help me deal with the crippling nausea. May 3 has always been the perfect time of year to me: The yard is bursting with signs of spring, and it's warm but not hot or humid. In the air you smell the respite from a long, cold winter, and the time is filled with hope. But on May 3, 2008, I don't see any of the hope, any of the promise. Sure my den chair sits beside the French doors that open into our backyard, and my two small kids scamper in and out of those doors at least a hundred times a day. Most of the time they beg me to come with them, to look at the gardenia bush about to bloom or to check out the cool bubble launcher their grandmother has brought them. Each time, I tell them I'll join them in a minute, never intending to make good on the promise. Eventually they stop asking, and I'm left to sit in the recliner, watching movies on Lifetime, dozing in and out of the fog of painkillers, listening to my children's laughter as they play outside.

Mom is visiting for my birthday, and she tries several times to talk me into coming out into the backyard to enjoy the day. I don't even try to fake it with her; I tell her I don't feel like it and that it should be my choice how I spend my birthday. She eventually gives up, too. Michael doesn't even really try. He's spent the last week or so working to get me out of my funk, to no avail. He is done. My husband, my mom, and my kids celebrate my birthday without me.

It has been about seven weeks since my gastric bypass surgery. I should be well on my way to finding a new normal in terms of how to eat. But the complications have set me back, both physically and psychologically. Here I am almost two months out, and I'm barely consuming two hundred calories a day. Nothing tastes right. Nothing sounds good. And I don't even want to deal with it, so I usually just don't. Because of that, I'm not getting any better. My body is weak and malnourished, and my soul needs feeding like nobody's business. I desperately need to know that one day I will feel better again, but no matter how many times my family and friends try to tell me that, I can't hear it. I won't believe it. I am as miserable as I've ever been.

∾

I was constantly reminded of what bad shape my body was in. My muscles were so weak, I quickly learned to avoid steps. Our sunken den only has two steps into the kitchen, but in order to climb them, I had to hang on to the wall and go one at a time. Once, I decided a soak in the tub sounded nice, and it did feel good, until I realized I couldn't climb out of it! I was unable to put my weight on my legs and pull myself out. Imagine my embarrassment when I had to call Michael in to help me.

My wounds from the gastric bypass had long healed, and my recovery from the complications should have been concluded. But my reliance on prescription pain medicine was as heightened as ever. I took those pills around the clock. If I missed a dose, I became antsy until I got my medication. I began to rely upon, and actually look forward to, the familiar haze that descended on me once the pills kicked in. My failures weren't quite so clear. My doubts weren't quite so real. I could deal with taking care of the kids and doing my job and going about all the mundane tasks we all have to each day, even when our very world is coming apart at the seams. The medication got me through each day . . . and I knew it was wrong. I knew there was no physical reason to continue taking painkillers; my body no longer ached. I was also constantly reminded about the toll the medication was taking on my body; the pills made me terribly nauseous, and the Zofran my doctor had prescribed no longer helped. I felt sick most of the time, but I didn't want to stop taking the Percocet. I told my doctor about the nausea and just let him assume it was left over from my surgery. He prescribed a nausea patch, and it worked wonders. I could now take the pain medicine and not feel so sick. I also knew, deep down, this was not a good thing, but I didn't want to stop. At that point it was the only thing that made me feel any better, the only way I felt anything even close to joy.

I had been warned about the potential pitfalls of post–gastric bypass surgery. Most of the time people overeat for a reason, and once they are physically unable to do so, they often find other forms of destructive behavior. Some become alcoholics, some develop gambling problems, others abuse drugs or cheat on their spouses. I knew that I was trying to find something to fill the void that food used to fill for me, but this was new territory. I had always thought of my overeating as a way to self-destruct. It never occurred to me that I also used food to cope, to bring about relief or happiness, even if it was just for the short term. Once bingeing wasn't an option for me, it became very clear that food had also served as a coping mechanism, and I was desperate to find something to take its place. As much as I didn't want to admit it, as much as it made me feel like the biggest cliché in the world, I started to realize that I was using prescription pain medicine to make me feel better.

Because I work in the news industry, I know the desperate lengths people will go to in order to get their hands on drugs. Stealing prescription pads, calling in phony orders to pharmacies, rummaging through the medicine cabinets of sick relatives—I knew several different (illegal) ways in which I could get more pills. It also occurred to me that I could probably get them by simply asking my doctor; hadn't I been through a lot? Would it be a big stretch to go to my surgeon and tell him I was still feeling pain and needed more medicine? I probably would have been able to pull it off, but I started to feel guilty about what I was doing. Taking the medicine and being in a constant fog was one thing; lying or at least stretching the truth to get more pills would mean I really had a problem. I was already trying to get rid of one heck of an addiction—did I really need another? No, I decided that if I went to extraordinary methods to get more pills, it would only mean that I was becoming reliant on the medicine, and I didn't need one more problem to get over. I still had plenty on my plate.

Of course this brave decision was easily made knowing what was waiting for me in my medicine cabinet. Having had two C-sections, I had a stash of painkillers left over from those surgeries. It's funny—I hadn't wanted to take those painkillers after giving birth because I thought they were bad news, and I didn't want to become dependent on them. I suppose that's an easy goal to carry out when you have a pretty newborn to take care of. Now it was just me, and I was miserable. I knew I didn't have to ask my doctor for more medicine because I already had some. Of course, I had a plan: I figured that as soon as those pills ran out, I would have to find my way around without them. Problem solved!

Some things never change.

I did stop taking the pills around the clock, just not completely; I knew that I could never get back to any sort of regular routine if I was doped up all the time. Slowly a skeleton of a life started to emerge. I got up in the morning and did my radio newscasts. I dressed the kids and took them to preschool. I worked during the day and did the bare minimum required to keep the house running. I picked up the kids from school, gave them a snack, and put them down for their naps. Then I took two pills and spent the rest of the afternoon zonked, sitting in my old chair with my table for my fan and my meds—unattached to my world and not feeling much of anything. It was nice; it felt good. And I justified it by telling myself I only did it once a day, that I was slowly getting better. I didn't return phone calls from friends. I avoided talking much to family members, other than the perfunctory "I'm fine" answers to their inquiries. I barely paid attention to my children. I just got through each day with the bare minimum. It was all I was capable of doing.

This went on for several weeks, and then Michael let me know he was sick of it. He knew I was taking Percocet and told me outright I should stop. I agreed, but then I ignored his pleas. I needed something to make me feel good, to make it seem as though everything was going to be okay. I still couldn't eat, and I was scared to try. I felt so abnormal and just . . . sick. The pills were the only thing that made it better.

I knew the medication was not a long-term solution, and I did want to find a way to get back to normal. I knew in my heart that not eating was no way to live; somehow I would have to find a way to find foods that I liked and could hold down. Before then I was too sick and too tired to take on what seemed like a monumental task; now I knew that the only way to recovery was to start nourishing my body.

And so it was almost two-and-a-half months after my surgery that I set about trying to eat. It was ridiculous that it took me that long, I know, but when I was feeling generous, I told myself that I'd been through a hard time and it was understandable. When I was beating myself up, I thought of how I could never do anything the "normal" way; there always had to be a glitch, some sort of obstacle to overcome. Still, I was finally determined to find a way to eat and feel better.

At first I decided it was best to buy what had been my favorite foods and just eat smaller portions. I went to my old favorite barbecue place and got a plate of vinegar-based barbecue, french fries, and hush puppies. I thought the barbecue would provide good protein, and I could just eat a couple of fries, just to satisfy my taste buds. After all, if I had a dollar for every french fry I'd eaten in my lifetime, I was sure I could find my place on the *Forbes* moneymakers list. I actually thought this fried-filled meal was a good first attempt.

Seeing all that food laid out on my plate made me want to hurl into oblivion. I tried the pork, ate two bites, and pushed away the plate. I thought maybe I could eat it later, but it was waiting for Michael when he came home, otherwise untouched. Back in my prime bingeing days, such a meal would have been merely a snack—an appetizer to a day's worth of gorging. Now I couldn't even stomach the idea of eating a third of the plate.

There were many other such attempts. I bought some spaghetti and meatballs from my favorite Italian place. I knew carbs were a big no-no for gastric bypass patients, but I figured I would eat mostly meat and some pasta. I couldn't even eat one whole meatball—more food left untouched. I went to a fast-food place and bought one single hamburger, thinking I could ditch the bun and just eat the patty. I barely ate half. And french fries? Ugh . . . they were so greasy and unappealing, I couldn't even bother. What a weird, new experience.

I slowly found things I could keep down. Mashed potatoes. Eggs. Cheese. I craved all kinds of high-carb foods, and I would go out and buy them, only to leave them virtually untouched. I guess it's true: The body does crave what it doesn't get, even if it can't tolerate it.

I learned this lesson with Doritos. I like the chips just as much as the next person, but I was never a huge fan before I had the surgery—I never went out of my way to eat them. But a few months after the gastric bypass, I found myself craving those nacho-flavored triangles. Again, I knew they were too high in carbs and too spicy for me, but I decided I had to have them anyway. I bought an individual bag and took them home. Michael was in the den with the kids, and I went into our bedroom with the Doritos and locked the door, as if I were doing something bad, or at least, something I knew I shouldn't be doing. I ate one chip. It tasted heavenly. I ate another, and another, and another. The flavors were so good, my taste buds were rejoicing. I guess all the dull foods I'd eaten for so long were getting kind of tiresome; I wanted flavor! I kept eating and eating, and soon I'd finished the entire bag. As I crunched on the last chip, a feeling of foreboding washed over me. What had I done? Was I crazy? I couldn't eat a whole bag of chips, even a small bag! What was going to happen to me? As I wiped my mouth, I waited.

I became so, so sick. Not the throwing up kind of sick; actually, that would have provided some sort of relief, I think. No, my belly just ached, and it was quite clear my body could not tolerate so many carbs, no matter how good they tasted. I disgustedly threw the bag in the trash and vowed never to eat them again.

Until the next day. Yes, the very next day. I remembered how flavorful the chips were and longed for that taste again. I bought another bag, promising myself this time I would not eat the whole thing. And I didn't; instead I ate only three-fourths of the bag. And once again I was so very sick, and just disgusted with myself. What had I expected? Was I a complete moron?

This happened several more times, with several different types of high-carb foods, before my mind finally got the message that my body was so desperately trying to convey: I can't eat a lot of carbs! They make me sick! As this realization finally sunk in, I couldn't help but shake my head at how long it took for me to learn the lesson, and then I had an epiphany: That's what it means to be a food addict. You know you are hurting yourself. You know what you are doing is not good. And you do it anyway. Over and over again. Because I had the gastric bypass surgery, I was finally physically unable to carry out my food addiction tendencies. But that didn't mean I didn't still want to, that I wouldn't try to. The instincts were still there, the drive to self-destruct was very much alive. And now that I was learning that I couldn't do it with food, I was looking for other ways to self-sabotage.

This realization helped me stop taking the Percocet. Well, to be honest, I ran out of the bottle left over from my second C-section, and I couldn't find the bottle from my first. I wasn't quite desperate enough to try lying to my doctor or breaking the law in order to keep the pill habit going, thank God. I did, however, turn the house upside down, looking for that other bottle of pills. I am so grateful that I never found them; another bottle's worth and I may have had another addiction on my hands. I realize that it could have happened, just like that.

I slowly started to put my life back together. I gave up sleeping in the recliner, and I put the Lego table that had become my portable medicine cabinet back in Eli's room. I finally returned phone calls and started catching up with all the friends who had been so worried about me. Of course they all understood that I had been through a lot, and they didn't hold any grudges; all they cared about was that I was okay. And I was starting to actually feel okay with going out in public. For the many weeks after the surgery and subsequent hospital stays, I avoided public situations as much as possible. I took the kids to preschool as early as I could, and I picked them up early in order to avoid the other moms. I stopped going to church. I even withdrew Emma from her ballet class. Every time I had to go out, I felt all eyes were on me, and I knew that most of the curiosity was truly out of concern. Everyone had heard what a hard time I was having, and they wanted to know if I was okay. But I felt so self-conscious, like such a freak, that I wanted to avoid public scrutiny as much as possible. I turned down playdate invitations, and I feigned excuses to miss birthday parties. My kids and I were holed up in my house, with me unable to deal with any kind of social pressure.

I knew that in order to return to any semblance of normalcy, I would have to slowly reintegrate myself into the mommy world. And it started at the end of May, when Emma's preschool class hosted a Muffins for Mom event. The kids were working so hard to put on this party for the class moms, I knew I had to go, even if I didn't feel quite up to seeing everyone. Figuring out what to wear, it occurred to me that this was the first time since the surgery I had really contemplated my appearance. I had been so caught up with being sick, and trying to figure out what to eat, I hadn't stopped to consider my weight. I was even still wearing my presurgery clothes; the baggy shirts and stretch pants fit perfectly with my mood. Of course I knew I'd lost weight; you can't go for two months without eating without losing some pounds. But I had no idea how much I'd lost, or how my body was adjusting.

I stepped on the scale, naked—278 pounds. In almost two and a half months, I'd lost close to sixty pounds. The very thought took my breath away. I remembered all the times I had struggled to lose even five pounds, all the effort it took to get through even one day without giving in to the urge to binge eat. It had been weeks and weeks since I felt the need to destroy myself with food, since I had stuffed myself so much that I thought I would vomit. When I stopped to consider that, I felt incredible relief. Yes, the past two months had been really, really hard—much more than I'd ever bargained for. But I was finally starting to see a bit of the sun, and knowing that the storm cloud of food addiction wasn't hanging over my head made me feel as though I could do anything. I felt free.

I went to the Muffins for Mom event in a black sweater that I hadn't worn in two years. Yes, I was still wearing black, and yes, I was still closer to three hundred pounds than I liked to be, but for the first time in a very, very long time, I felt I was moving in the right direction. The other moms greeted me warmly, all concerned about how I was doing and all commenting on how good I looked. More than one person said I was starting to get my color back. I knew what they were talking about. I was starting, ever so slowly, to feel like myself again. Not the bloated, out-of-control eating self. And not the sickly, pill-reliant woman I had threatened to become. I was finally starting to feel like just Jennifer. And that was finally starting to feel like it was enough.

13

Finally, the Dawn

OCTOBER 2008

I'm at the Pumpkin Patch with my four-year-old daughter's preschool class. Even though we are surrounded by bales of hay, barrels of red apples, and stacks and stacks of bright orange pumpkins, the air is warm on my cheeks and all I can think about is spring. Several months before, after my gastric bypass surgery, I missed the birth of spring; because of the complications, I hardly noticed the pink blooming azaleas or the grass turning from brown straw into a rich field of green. But now, in this moment of my life, it feels like springtime. Hope renewed. A rebirthing, if you will.

Emma has a classmate named Will-Parks, a cute little blond boy she's known since they were babies. I tell her all the time that Will-Parks's daddy is a hero—he's a soldier stationed at Fort Bragg, and we've watched him deploy overseas several times over the years. I've always admired the way his mother cares for her children while her husband is away, seemingly with such ease. I can't imagine having that kind of strength. I've also enjoyed watching Will-Parks's dad over the years when he is home, because he is such a loving, doting father. All the kids in Emma's preschool class love him.

On this day, Will-Parks's dad approaches me as we wait for the slideshow to begin in the farmhouse. The kids are happily munching on homemade ice cream, and he leans over to get my attention. I smile warmly at him; it has been a while since we've seen each other. He's tentative, which is kind of unusual for him. Finally, he says, "I . . . I hope it's okay. Can I say . . . can I tell you . . . how great you look?"

If my smile were any bigger, my face would be permanently disfigured.

He's instantly relieved that I'm not embarrassed or offended, and this makes me admire him even more. It's scary for a man to say anything even remotely related to weight to a woman; I've definitely learned that over the years. He got past that because he thought it was important that I hear what he had to say, and I am so grateful that he did. Women do need to hear compliments, especially from dashing, good-looking soldiers. I needed to hear a wonderfully warm compliment, unsolicited.

Take that, sun god Scott.

෴

I lost one hundred pounds in six months. Just writing that statement is mind-blowing; living it has been an unbelievable whirlwind. I can't tell you how much I dreamed over the years of losing one hundred pounds, how many different plans and schemes I hatched trying to reach that goal, only to fail time and again. To finally have it happen, to finally be out of the morbidly obese category is something I find difficult to describe. Joy. Relief. Freedom. Those are the words that come to mind.

Anyone who thinks having gastric bypass surgery is taking the easy way out really needs to come and live my life, from the beginning, on March 18, when I was rolled out of the OR in such pain and it took months to recover. I did finally get over the physical pain, and I am making strides in the psychological arena as well. But make no mistake: No part of this has been easy—not even close.

I sometimes wonder if I will ever eat "normally" again. And I guess I should figure out how I define normal; certainly how I ate before the surgery wouldn't qualify. I guess my question is . . . will I ever blend in? Will people ever stop taking account of what I'm eating or asking me about what foods I should avoid? Will I ever be able to take a trip again without some elaborate plan to have foods that I can tolerate? Really, I'm dying to know how this will all play out.

For now, I am getting nourishment daily, and that is certainly progress. The crippling nausea is gone, thank goodness, and I have a pretty good idea of what foods agree with me and which ones I should avoid. Despite my best efforts, I still get in too big of a hurry sometimes, and I don't chew my food thoroughly. When this happens, food gets stuck in my esophagus, and I have to remind myself first of all to stay calm. Usually I then get out my familiar green bowl. It's become known affectionately in my house as "Mommy's throw-up bucket." When my food gets stuck, I have to get it out the old-fashioned way. I have thrown up more in the last year than I have my entire life. It's such a regular occurrence, my children don't even notice it anymore. It used to be quite upsetting, and I'll admit, it still isn't my favorite thing in the world. But I've learned to live with it, and I am convinced it is getting better. My stomach pouch will stretch over time, and as I continue to learn what foods to cut out, I'm sure much progress will be made.

The number one question I get is, "What do you eat?" Indeed, everyone is so curious about me at mealtime, it's kind of amusing. I know a couple of people who had a gastric bypass who resent this kind of attention. But really, I don't mind it at all. I understand it, in fact; I've always been deeply curious about how all this works. I just worry that I am not a model patient and perhaps not the best example of what to do and what not to do! In any case, protein is the order of the day. Now that I finally have gotten the message that carbs are not my friend, I eat very few of them. It was never my intention to cut out carbs entirely; they just don't agree with my stomach. So I don't eat sandwiches or pasta or potatoes. Well, I guess that is not entirely true; I will eat a bite of spaghetti or a french fry or two. But truly, I've lost my taste for high-carb foods, and I couldn't be more grateful. Besides, I've eaten enough plates of spaghetti to last me a lifetime!

I have two scrambled eggs every morning, usually with some cheese. For snacks, I eat slices of pepperoni or table-spoons of peanut butter or a handful of nuts. I still enjoy lean red meats, but I have trouble tolerating hamburger, and I still haven't found any chicken that I enjoy—something about it is too chewy for me. Really, if it weren't for cheese, I wouldn't survive!

Of course, the one million dollar question is: What do I drink? Have I fared well with the no-soft-drinks rule? The relief-filled answer is an easy yes. Truly, it was the one thing I was most worried about, and it is actually what I have missed the least. Maybe in that way, the complications after my surgery were a blessing; I was too preoccupied with illness to obsess over my inability to have a Coke. And I found that once I didn't have them often, I didn't miss them—not at all. I've had conversations with other gastric bypass patients who've tried to tell me it would be all right to have a drink every once in a while, but I am not going there. I've been through too much to risk it, thank you very much.

In fact during the 2008 Christmas season, I took my daughter to a cookie exchange at a girlfriend's house. The moms hosting the event thought it would be cute to make Shirley Temples for the little girls to drink. I guess I'm an idiot—I had no idea what was in a Shirley Temple. When they handed me Emma's pink drink, I sipped some off the top so she wouldn't spill it all over herself. I immediately tasted the carbonation and almost spit the drink out all over the table! I didn't realize Shirley Temples are made with Sprite. Truly, it tasted awful, and Michael has said the same. He gave up soft drinks the same time I did, although every once in a while he gets served one by mistake. He says when you're not used to it, the carbonation is dreadful. I'll just take his word for it. Other than that one sip, I haven't had a soda since March 17, 2008, and I don't plan to ever have one again.

It doesn't mean I've said good-bye to sweet drinks, however. After the surgery, I had a huge problem with dehydration, but water just didn't do it for me. I needed to find something that I would drink regularly—and I turned at first to my kids' juice boxes. I loved the sweet taste, and the small amounts were just what I needed. Of course they had too much sugar in them, and I'm sure my surgeon would frown about me drinking them. Again, I don't claim to be a model patient; I just had to do whatever it took at the time. I did eventually give them up—but for pleasure, I now turn to the wine of the south, sweet tea. It gives me the sweet taste without the carbonation of soda. Yes, it is full of sugar and calories and not the best thing in the world for me. But I like it, and I allow it, and that's all I'm going to say about it (believe me, I get plenty of grief from Michael).

Something I've taken great pleasure in is my absolute indifference to fast food. I used to live in the drive-thru line, and now I couldn't care less about it. The only reason I ever go at all is if my children want the latest kid's meal toy; I rarely get anything to eat for myself. I find most of the food too greasy and it upsets my stomach. What a victory this is! Although I must admit that it is not terribly convenient. If I'm out and about and have to find something to eat, it makes things a little trickier. I always have the need to plan in advance, but really, that's only a small nuisance. The fact that I can pass all those fast-food signs and keep right on driving is thrilling.

Another mild irritation that comes as a result of having a gastric bypass is not being able to drink with my meals. To allow room in my stomach pouch for my food, I have to stop drinking anything thirty minutes before I eat, and I have to wait to have something to drink for at least thirty minutes after I eat. I knew this before the surgery, and I thought of all the changes I would have to make, this would be the least bothersome. But it has actually turned out to be the toughest to get used to. I mean, it's just natural to want to sip something while you eat, especially when you eat things like cheese and peanut butter! But I've really had to train myself not to, and I'm getting there. When I go to restaurants, I purposefully don't order anything, because even if it's just water, I will pick it up and drink it out of habit. Drinking while eating makes eating really uncomfortable, so I'm learning to avoid it, albeit reluctantly.

I am so very happy to report that my diabetes has gone away, as has my high blood pressure. I can't tell you what a tremendous relief this is; being diagnosed with type 2 diabetes after Eli was born really put me over the edge. The thought of being on medication, and possibly on insulin shots, for the rest of my life was unfathomable. Getting rid of those two conditions alone was worth having the surgery, even with all its complications.

I do struggle with vitamin deficiency, as most gastric bypass patients do. The way my body absorbs vitamins from food has been changed forever, and I will always be on supplements. I take multivitamins twice a day, plus a calcium supplement. And after having recent blood work, my surgeon has me on a vitamin D supplement. I hate having to take pills every day, but it's a small price to pay; I've learned not to take good health for granted.

In fact, it was the vitamin deficiency aspect of all of this that led to perhaps one of the worst postsurgery complications, at least for personal reasons.

I lost a lot of hair. Now, it's well-known that this is a common side effect for gastric bypass patients; after the surgery your body is in such shock that every available vitamin and nutrient goes to support your major organs and body systems, and things such as hair, skin, and nails miss out. It's not uncommon for gastric bypass patients to go through quite a bit of "shedding"— and doctors advise their patients not to be alarmed, the hair will come back. But if you'll recall, I'd been going through hair loss for quite some time leading up to the surgery. For years I'd been self-conscious about my protruding scalp, wondering if everyone else noticed that my hair was thinning. I was warned about this side effect before the surgery, but I guess I didn't seriously contemplate the ramifications. I just wanted the weight off, no matter what it took. But about three months post-op, once the complications were finally behind me and I was starting to live again, I started to lose gobs and gobs of hair. It was frightening. My previous hair loss was way more subtle—a few strands in the shower, on my clothes, and so on. This time fistfuls would drop into my hairbrush every morning. I'd find tangles of hair in the washing machine from my clothes. I was shedding everywhere: on the carpet, in the car, on the plate of food at the dinner table. More than once two-year-old Eli came to me, saying, "Mommy hair in my mouth." It was humiliating, and it did a real number on my self-confidence.

Had I really come all this way, only to look like a complete freak? Sure, I was losing weight, but how would anyone notice? They'd be too busy staring at my bald scalp! I tried to comb it and style it in a way that hid what was happening, but truly, each day, I was so scared to look in the mirror, afraid to see even more hair gone. I didn't know what to do.

When I went in for my sixth-month checkup, the hair loss was the only concern I brought up to the doctor. He nodded and said it was quite common, and that it would grow back, perhaps even thicker and fuller—all the things I'd read. Only, I'd suffered hair loss before the surgery—would my situation be different? Did that mean my hair would not come back? The doctor didn't know—he'd never been asked that question. I was as confused and scared as ever.

I seriously started to think about getting a wig. I was becoming so self-conscious; I didn't want to leave the house. That was frightening, considering I was just rebounding from the surgery complications and depression. I couldn't believe I found myself wanting to hide again. Maybe a wig would make me more comfortable; after all, they make really good ones now, in all kinds of styles. They are quite realistic looking. And maybe I wouldn't have to wear it for long; if what the doctor said was true, my hair would come back. Perhaps a wig was what I needed to get through the interim.

I started researching and found that wigs are very, very expensive. If I wanted one that was going to fool people, and indeed I did, it would cost me at least a thousand dollars. I struggled with this. On the one hand, I thought it would do me a lot of good in terms of self-confidence. But on the other hand, we had a lot of medical bills to pay, plus we weren't exactly rich to begin with. Could I justify spending so much money on something I was truly hoping was only temporary?

While I was mulling it over, I decided to share what I was going through with some friends. Whenever someone asked how I was doing, or remarked on how great I looked, I thanked them and admitted that my only problem was my hair. Most people seemed concerned, and I explained how the doctor had said it was only temporary. Everywhere I turned, I received kind words and encouragement, and in the end, I decided not to invest in the wig. I figured if I suddenly showed up with a full head of hair, everyone would know it wasn't real, and that would instantly cause talk and speculation. What was the point? By being open and upfront about the problem, I found myself liberated from being so self-conscious about it. Instead of letting it control me, I took control of it. That felt wonderful.

I am happy to report that my hair is coming back, albeit slowly. I have tiny little hairs standing straight up all over my scalp. Yes, it looks freaky, but I don't care. I love every single hair, and I gleefully point them out to anyone and everyone who asks how I am doing!

There have been many victories to enjoy so far on this path. The very last week of May, as I was just beginning to come out of the post-op complication fog, we took our kids to the beach for a weekend trip. Normally I'd rejoice in the timing of the excursion; late May is usually too cold to get in any kind of water for very long, and as a fat person, I could easily be excused for not putting on a bathing suit. Even though I'd had gastric bypass surgery and was on my way to a healthier me, I was still quite heavy, and didn't relish the thought of going half-naked in public. But we were going to a resort with an indoor water park! Hooray! Bathing suit required! Shoot me now, right? Wrong. I planned the trip, on purpose, knowing what was involved. And I embraced it. Well, perhaps *embrace* is a little strong; it was still quite difficult for me to imagine wearing a bathing suit in front of a lot of people.

But something changes when you're headed down the scale instead of going up. The idea of taking a risk is somehow more tolerable, especially when it pertains to your kids having fun. I bought a Delta Burke bathing suit, in black. It was a size 2X and had a little skirt on it for extra coverage. But by God, it was a bathing suit and I wore it. I swam with my kids, for hours on end, listening to their laughter and glee. Every time I had to get out of the water, I felt as though everyone was staring at me. I fantasized about calling everyone's attention to announce that, yes, I was heavy, but just so they knew, I was finally doing something about it. I didn't want everyone to take one look at the miserably fat woman in the bathing suit and feel sorry for me. When I dwelled on stuff like that, I was a little down. But I knew next summer would be different, and the next and the next. And that felt priceless.

Later that summer we actually joined a pool. I had wondered for years how my kids would get the privilege of swimming if I wasn't able to do it with them, and finally I was not only able but willing. I wore the same 2X bathing suit all summer, even after it was clearly too big for me. I was self-conscious at first, but after a while, I let it go. I was there for my kids to have fun, and I didn't care what strangers thought about me. I knew I was losing weight and getting healthier every day, and that was truly all that mattered. It was so liberating.

Over all the years I struggled with trying to lose weight, I would fantasize about all the clothes I was going to wear once I was thinner. As I gained weight and slowly grew out of all my thinner clothes, I held on to them like trophies, vowing one day I would wear them again. Old dresses, suits, and even jeans all hung in my closet, waiting to be worn again. Of course when I finally started to really shed the pounds, some sixteen years later, most of the clothes were grossly out of style. Acid-washed jeans, anyone? No, wearing my old clothes, for the most part, was not an option. But I was able to make it through the first several months postsurgery thanks to hand-me-downs from friends who had lost weight. My sister-in-law, Mandy, in particular, saved me thousands of dollars in clothes. She gave me tons of high-quality tops, pants, and dresses that started in size 2X and went down to size 16. For many months after the surgery, I didn't have to buy anything, and that was a good thing, too. Shopping now intimidated me greatly. I was woefully unprepared to look for clothes when there were lots of options to be had; I was used to having to settle on whatever I could find that would fit me. Suddenly I was faced with having lots and lots of styles and colors to choose from, and I had no idea what was hip and what kinds of clothes were flattering on me. I needed help, fast!

Things only got worse once I sized out of the "today's woman" category of clothing. The regular-size parts of the department store were so intimidating to me, I didn't know where to begin. I tried a few times to shop, and I swear I had panic attacks. My mind got swimmy, my heart beat fast, and I had to get the heck out of there. One time I was so scared, I retreated to the big woman's section and actually convinced myself that some 1X tops still fit me. When I put them on at home, my mom, who was visiting at the time, couldn't believe her eyes. Why had I bought such big shirts? Funny, to me they hadn't looked that big in the store, but she was right: They were way too big for me. Such a revelation should have made me happy, and it did, but I was also scared of the unknown. I hadn't bought regular clothes in more than a decade. I didn't know what in the world I was doing.

The weight loss was happening so fast, my mind had a hard time keeping up. The scales said one thing, but inside I felt the same. I knew I was thinner, but it was hard for me to believe I had lost so many pounds that I could now wear an extra-large instead of a 2X. To someone who's never battled a weight problem, this may not seem like much, but trust me, the difference is huge.

I walked around with baggy, ill-fitting clothes for a while. I knew I could do better, but I felt paralyzed. Finally a special occasion approached, and I needed a new outfit. Desperate, I went to a small department store with an even smaller ladies' department. The bigger woman sizes were smashed in right beside the normal clothes, and before I knew it, I had crossed the line and was looking at tops in 14, 16, and 18. I quickly drew in a breath, waiting for the panic attack to settle in. Surprisingly I remained calm. I looked for something I liked. I found it in a 16. I went to the dressing room. And . . . it fit! And it looked great. I couldn't believe it. Up until then, whenever I'd wandered into the regular-size section, I half expected someone to tap me on the shoulder, telling me I didn't belong. Finally, I knew I did.

I've had many people ask me about gastric bypass surgery. So many seem to know someone who they think would benefit from it, and they want to know if I recommend it. This is a tough one for me. On the one hand, I do not regret at all having had the surgery. Even though I had a lot of complications, and it certainly hasn't been an easy road, I know the path I had been on was one that led to premature death. That may sound overdramatic to some people, but please believe me: I was slowly killing myself with food. And what's worse, I knew that's what I was doing and was unable to stop myself. Finally making the decision to have a gastric bypass saved my life—I truly believe that. Was it fun to have the abscess, the collapsed lung, the depression? Of course not. But the way I was going, it wouldn't have been long before I suffered a stroke or a heart attack. I could have easily dropped dead, leaving a husband and two children behind to mourn what could have been. So yes, I am happy I had gastric bypass surgery and I would do it all over again.

Would I encourage others to do it? No. I just couldn't, not after what I went through. I endured months of pain and depression. I still don't know what the future holds in terms of side effects. But at least I know that I made this decision myself; I didn't let anyone else talk me into it. And that's what everyone else has to do, too. Before agreeing to have this surgery, you must really understand what it entails—and what could happen. And you have to be willing to live with the results. It takes a lot of research and soul-searching. I am happy to share my story with anyone who wants to listen. But such an important decision has to be made by the individual themselves.

As the weight has come off, I have given much thought to addiction and the ramifications of this hideous disease. For years I felt like a rat trapped in a cage. The harder I tried to get out, the more stuck I became. It occurs to me now that I couldn't really fix the problem since I didn't know what it was. Meaning, I bought into what society tells us about weight loss: Put in the hard work and you will see results. When you hit rock bottom, you will find your way back up. How many rock bottoms did I hit over the years? How many nights found me on my knees, begging God for answers? I thought I would find the solution with a new diet plan, a new exercise routine, or a new bottle of pills. I never really understood that the food and the weight gain were only symptoms—they were tools in my arsenal of self-destruction. Now that I've had weight-loss surgery, I have taken away my ability to hurt myself with food, and I thank God for that every day. But unfortunately, my desire to hurt myself has not entirely gone away.

At the same time that I was put back into the hospital with complications from the surgery, my mother was diagnosed with colorectal cancer. She kept her diagnosis from me for weeks, worried that I would turn my back on my recovery to focus on her. When she did finally tell me, I was scared to death. But we rallied as a family to see her through the treatment. She had six weeks of radiation and chemo, followed by surgery. After a week in the hospital, she was sent home to recover before another six months of chemotherapy. It was a scary and stressful time, and I stayed with her for her first few days at home. I had to go to the pharmacy to fill her bottle of Percocet. I laughed a little to myself as I purchased the one-hundred-count bottle of painkillers; hadn't I been frantically searching for these pills just months before? I was so glad they made me so sick, sure that I could have become addicted to them if they didn't. I gave my mom her medicine and started to cook dinner.

I couldn't stop thinking about the pills. I remembered how they took away the pain, and not just the physical pain. They helped me to not feel anything: the hurt, the feelings of failure after my surgery went wrong. I was so scared I had made a mistake, that I would never be normal again, and the pills helped me stuff all those problems away, much like food had. Being with my mom, seeing her in pain, and not knowing what the future held for her scared me to death. I'd lost my dad four years before; the thought of my mom dying was too much to bear. My mom had one hundred pills—she wouldn't notice if I took a couple, right? I just wanted a break, I wanted to feel good for a change.

Once I made the decision to do it, I felt giddy. It reminded me of how I felt once I finally relented and ate my brains out after a day of going back and forth with my demons. Once I was on my way to pick up the food, or in the drive-thru line, I felt relief, like I was getting away from crushing pain and guilt. This was much the same—ever since I'd picked up my mom's medicine, I wrestled with myself over trying them, just once. I knew it wasn't right, that I had no business taking those pills. But I finally decided to do it, and I was excited.

I ate first, trying to stave off nausea. I made sure my mom was all settled in for the night. And then I took two pills. I sat on the couch in front of the TV and waited. It was only about fifteen minutes before I was flying higher than a kite. I could feel the blood coursing through my veins, and the rush was terrific. I could almost see myself sitting there with a big, stupid smile on my face, and I was disgusted. *What in the world am I doing?* I thought to myself. I was the kid who never drank in high school, who never even tried smoking a joint. Now I was taking prescription painkillers recreationally? Just as the doubts started creeping in, the room started to spin a little. The familiar waves of nausea started to hit, and I felt so, so sick. I was hot and sweaty, and my heart was pounding. I lay down under the ceiling fan, trying to get cool, trying to calm down. I wanted to throw up so bad, but this kind of nausea isn't that kind—you're stuck at the point of wanting to vomit but not quite being able to. It was torture, and it went on for hours.

I finally passed out on the couch, and when I awoke the next day, I was still reeling. The thought of breakfast turned my stomach, and the room still spun as I made my way to take care of Mom. I felt so completely stupid for what I had done, and also suddenly very sober about the possibilities. What if I wasn't so sick? What if all I felt after taking that Percocet was the incredible high and that wonderful fog, removing me from reality and all its problems? I could have very easily become addicted to those pills, and I knew it. It scared the crap out of me. Suddenly it all made sense.

Something within me doesn't sit well with happiness. Things start going well, life is good, and the beast inside rears its ugly head. It used to be a destructive boyfriend. For many, many years, food was its weapon of choice. Now, it was dormant, but its heart was still clinging to life. The beast was looking for another tool to use against me, and I knew I was in trouble.

Thank God painkillers make me too sick to function. But what if something else destructive takes a liking to me? Alcohol, street drugs, gambling, overspending . . . there are a number of ways to ruin your life, if you're hell-bent on doing so. And apparently, I was. It scares me to death.

I went to my general practitioner and had an open and honest discussion about antidepressants. I told her I was having trouble dealing with stress and anxiety and felt I needed something to help me relieve the symptoms—something that was sanctioned by a doctor and not illegal or destructive. She asked me several questions about what I'd been feeling and what events led to those feelings. At the end of the talk, we agreed on which medication to try at a low dose. More important, she made me promise that I would not stop taking the meds without first talking with her and that I would be honest about how the pills were helping and how, if at all, they seemed to harm me. For the first time, I had a positive talk about using antidepressants, and I felt good about the possibility of taking something that I was now convinced I needed.

It took a couple of months of tweaking, but I definitely see a difference in how I feel each day and how I cope with everyday life. Is it all picnics and roses? No, and it never will be. But it is hopeful, and I haven't been able to say that in a really, really long time. It feels good.

For years I fought the suggestion of taking antidepressants, and now I feel silly for doing so. Admitting you need help is not admitting failure; it is actually a step toward success. And that's how I feel about having had gastric bypass surgery. After hearing my story I'm sure anyone would agree, it wasn't taking the easy way out, not by any stretch of the imagination. But agreeing to the procedure meant I was finally able to say, "You know what? I can't do this on my own—I need help." And taking that step was the bravest thing I could do for myself. I now know that to be true.

Not being under the crushing pressure of addiction is a high all its own. I don't obsess twenty-four hours a day about what I have eaten or what I will eat. I don't weigh myself every day; I rarely make it on the scale once a week. I haven't lost all of the weight I would like to lose, but that's okay. I know it will happen eventually, and in the meantime, I'm not worried about it. And that is incredibly freeing.

Our society doesn't take food addiction seriously. People who have never struggled with their weight look at the obese and think, "Why don't they just stop eating?" If only it were that simple! Trust me, no one chooses to be morbidly obese. I know there are a lot of people out there who sound the battle cry of "Big Is Beautiful." I'm here to tell them that "Big Is Deadly." Indeed, I think it is impossible for anyone to be truly happy if he or she is morbidly obese. Just the physical ramifications of carrying around so much weight prevent one from being able to enjoy life fully. Do I think all heavy people are as miserable as I was? Definitely not. Truly, I think so many people handle it way better than I ever did or could have. But if they are trying to fool others into thinking they are happy with being one hundred or more pounds over-weight, they are only fooling themselves. And I wish they could live one day in my shoes, to know that it doesn't have to be that way.

I go to restaurants and don't worry about being able to fit into the booth. I visit the movie theater and feel comfortable in its seats. I attend preschool functions and am fine sitting in the tiny chairs. I blend into the crowd, and I feel glorious. And sometimes, every once in a while, I even feel a little pretty.

I'm starting to love exercise again, but it took a long time. After the surgery and complications, I was in no mood to do anything physical. My muscles were so weak, I found simply climbing a flight of stairs exhausting. But slowly that changed. I started with ten minutes on the treadmill every day for a week. Then I increased it to fifteen, then twenty. I'm now up to forty-five minutes daily, and I find that on the days I don't exercise, I miss it. That feeling is so wonderful, to actually crave working out. One day, I vow to start running, like I've always dreamed of doing. This is the first time I've really thought it was possible.

Like most gastric bypass patients, excess skin is a problem. I find I have extra folds especially around my bra line, my abdomen, and my thighs. It is unsightly; I'm not going to lie. But am I upset enough to do something about it? The jury is still out on that one. My experiences in the hospital have left deep scars, and I'm not talking about the surgeries. Right now I'm still wary of all things medical; indeed, it took me months to agree to simply go have blood drawn for a physical. I never used to be scared of needles or doctors, but I must say I have some real phobias right now. Hopefully time and a little distance will alleviate those fears, and perhaps one day I'll look into having reconstructive surgery for my skin. But right now I'm just not there yet. And that's fine with me.

I don't remember getting below three hundred pounds; it happened when I was still sick and dealing with complications. I remember being vaguely happy about reaching that milestone, but with everything else that was going on, it was sort of anticlimactic. But I had months and months to think about getting below two hundred pounds. It was just another number, but I honestly couldn't wait for it to happen. As it turned out, I had to wait a long, long time. At first I thought I would easily reach it by Christmas of 2008. I fantasized about the family gathering and my showing up in a fabulous outfit, weighing less than two hundred pounds for the first holiday in more than fifteen years. But as December 25 approached, and I hovered around 214, it began to look like it wasn't going to happen. I had a brief moment of panic . . . and I started to plan in a frenzy: If I skipped some meals, cut down to low-fat cheese, amped up my exercise, maybe, possibly, I could . . . wait. I stopped myself cold. The three seconds that I allowed myself to think that way turned me back into a person I never wanted to be again. Unrealistic plans, desperate attempts at fast weight loss. Those days were behind me. They were just numbers on a scale. Whether I was 214 pounds or 198 pounds on Christmas Day, I was going to look fabulous, and feel even better. Nothing else mattered.

I did get below two hundred pounds, in February 2009, and I did mark the occasion . . . with a little naked dance in my bathroom, alone. And then I went right on my way. They were just numbers, and I didn't need a scale to tell me how I felt.

My husband and I went out to celebrate our sixteenth wedding anniversary, and for once I had unlimited choices in what to wear. I spent the evening not obsessing over everything on my plate. Instead I enjoyed talking with Michael without the distraction of food or self-loathing. Finally I'm able to appreciate all my many blessings: a wonderful marriage, two great, healthy kids, and finally, some happiness. I will never, ever take it for granted again.

I look at the many, many people struggling with the same problems I did for years, and I pray for them. I really want to reach out to those folks, to tell them my story and how it doesn't have to be this way, but alas, that is not allowed. I can't approach someone I don't know and have a conversation with him or her about his or her weight; if that had happened to me, I would have died of embarrassment and humiliation on the spot. And I also don't think that every overweight person out there is a food addict. Indeed for years I struggled with my weight, but I wasn't addicted to food; it wasn't until I began using food as a weapon against myself, getting caught in the cycle of binge and regret, that I truly had a problem. Just because someone is heavy doesn't mean he or she can't stop being so on his or her own. But I do know that there are many people out there suffering as I did all those years. They try and do the right thing, but they are stuck—unable to break the cycle. My heart aches for them, and I want them to know they are not alone. And they are not worthless. The medical community has to do a better job of helping people with food addiction. And our society needs to recognize that this is a very serious illness, one that can have deadly consequences. It's only when we truly understand a problem that we can begin to solve it.

I've learned to live my life not for the big, earth-shattering events that I have fantasized about all of my life, but instead for the small victories that occur along my daily path. Like the day, seven months after my gastric bypass surgery, I was able to wear my wedding rings again. They hadn't fit for years, and I'd longed for the day that I would finally be able to put them back on. Emma, at four-and-a-half-years old, had never seen the rings before; I hadn't been able to wear the set since way before she was born. "Mommy!" she gasped, grabbing my hand. "You look like a princess!"

I smiled down at her, gazing at my diamonds. And then I caught a glimpse of myself in the mirror. My daughter thought I looked like a princess. And finally, looking at my reflection and actually liking what I saw, I was beginning to feel like one, too.

Acknowledgments

I would like to thank my husband, Michael, for his unlimited love and support—of me and, in particular, of this book. Thanks for listening when I asked, pushing when I needed it, and shouldering all the parenting duties when I needed to take the day to write. I've thought from the beginning that God Himself planted you in my path, and you've proven my theory correct over and over again. I love you.

To Mom: Thanks for being my cheerleader and helping me believe I could do anything I set my mind to. I've never met a more selfless person, and I hope I am able to give my children as much love as you have shown me. You are the best.

To my agent, Kathy Green: This book would not have happened without you. Thank you for taking a chance on me and believing that I had something valuable to say. Your support has been a godsend.

To the folks at Globe Pequot Press, especially Kristen Mellitt, and, in particular, Lara Asher: I still don't know how I got so lucky to have you on this book and in my life. Your contributions have made my story so much better, and your enthusiasm has meant the world to me. I thank you so very much.

To the folks at WRAL-TV and Capitol Broadcasting: Thank you for being such a wonderful work family.

To Deb Happel: Thank you for volunteering your editing services when I first started this book—your input was invaluable.

To Amanda Lamb: Thank you for laying out the blueprint for me, and for all the advice and support that went with it.

To David McCorkle: Thank you for being willing to help me, even when I didn't know what it was I needed. You helped me find the way.

To Julia Milstead, Melissa Buscher, Mandy Brown, and Jennifer Christiansen: Thanks for being willing to listen when even I was sick of hearing it. Your friendship got me through.

I have the three best sisters-in-law in the world. Thank you to Carol Anne Fry for encouragement and expert photo-taking; Molly Joyner for always being willing to be my sounding board while I try to work things out; and Mandy King, for daring to pose the question that made me take action. It quite simply saved my life.

And to all my family: Thank you for allowing me to share my story and your parts in it. I love you all.

About the Author

Jennifer Joyner is a journalist with more than sixteen years' experience covering the news in North and South Carolina. In her career she has worn many hats: television reporter, morning radio show cohost, news director, and featured writer. For the past ten years, home for Jennifer has been WRAL-TV, one of the largest CBS affiliates in the country. For WRAL, she helps gather news for the Raleigh/Durham/Fayetteville markets. She also anchors morning newscasts for two radio stations in Fayetteville, one of which, WZFX-FM, is one of the most dominant urban radio stations in the southeastern United States. Jennifer is also a featured writer for WRAL.com and chronicles her personal journey at jenniferjoyner.com.

Jennifer has been married to her husband, Michael, a news photographer for WRAL-TV, for seventeen years. They have two children—Emma is six, and Eli is five. They make their home in Fayetteville, North Carolina.